CARING FOR YOUR SICK

CAT

with 70 Photographs

Carol Himsel Daly, DVM

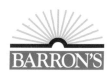

BARRON'S

Dedication

This book is dedicated with affection to Katherine West, devoted friend and quintessential care-giver to all species.

© Copyright 1994 by Barron's Educational Series, Inc.

All inquiries should be addressed to:
Barron's Educational Series, Inc.
250 Wireless Boulevard
Hauppauge, New York 11788

International Standard Book No. 0-8120-1726-9

Library of Congress Catalog Card No. 93-43105

Library of Congress Cataloging-in-Publication Data

Himsel Daly, Carol.
     Caring for your sick cat / Carol Himsel Daly.
         p.   cm.
     Includes bibliographical references and index.
     ISBN 0-8120-1726-9
     1. Cats—Diseases—Nursing. 2. Cats—Wounds and injuries—Treatment. 3. Care of sick animals. 4. Veterinarian and client. I. Title.
SF 985.H644   1994
636.8'089—dc20   93-43105
                                                                    CIP

PRINTED IN HONG KONG

67   9927   98765432

Photo credits: Most of the photographs in this book were taken by the author or by Don Himsel of Advantage Communications. The photographs appearing on the following pages were taken by Susan Green: pages 40, 67, 68, 79, 91; Donna Coss: page 104; Brian Blauser: page 159; Phil Maggitti: page 87. The photographs on the inside covers were taken by Donna Coss.

About the author: After practicing for several years in northern California, Dr. Carol Himsel Daly currently resides with her husband Richard on the Connecticut shoreline where she practices veterinary medicine and surgery for small companion animals. In addition, Dr. Himsel is a veterinary consultant and has written research and clinical articles for the scientific community. She is also the author of *Rats—A Complete Pet Owner's Manual* (Barron's). When she is not caring for other peoples' animals, Dr. Himsel spends her time caring for Willie, Neige, Cocoa and Molly and dabbles in the arts of photography and cooking.

Important Note: When you handle cats you may sometimes get scratched or bitten. if this happens, have a doctor treat the injuries immediately.

Make sure your cat receives all the necessary shots and wormings, otherwise serious danger to the animal and to human health may arise. A few diseases and parasites can be communicated to humans. If your cat shows any signs of illness, you should definitely consult a veterinarian. If you are worried about your own health, see your doctor and tell him or her that you have cats.

Some people have allergic reactions to cat hair. If you think you might be allergic, ask your doctor before you get a cat.

It is possible for a cat to cause damage to someone else's property and even to cause accidents. For your own protection you should make sure your insurance covers such eventualities, and you should definitely have liability insurance.

Contents

Part II THE CONVALESCENT CAT

Introduction

Whiskers, Woody, Wheezer, Willie, Nilly, Nicky, Nix-Nooks, Spooky, Sam, Dazzy, Dozer, Zebra, Zack, Zoom, Moe, Megan, Paddy-O, Prince, Pasha, Tosca, Timmy, Toes, Rose, Ripper, Rusty, Ralph, and Fred came to see me on Thursday. Most everybody needed a vaccination and a checkup to make sure everything was okay. Prince came in a box, and he was royally upset about it too. Rusty's foot was sore—he fell off the roof last night. Wheezer turned her nose up at her favorite food again that day, so her mistress was worried. Zack is on a diet; he comes once a month for a weigh-in and moral support. Ralph didn't need anything, but he came along with Fred, just because. And everybody had more fleas than necessary.

During my practice of veterinary medicine over the last nine years, I've been fortunate to have clients who, for the most part, follow my instructions about vaccinations, medication, exercise, diet, and reexamination as best they can. Often, our pet owners leave late for work, ask a friendly neighbor to check in, take the day off, or even cancel a vacation to see that their beloved companion is comfortable, and that medication is given on time. For their efforts, preventable diseases aren't often a problem, and kitties like Rusty once more prowl the roof.

Many people go farther and commit themselves emotionally and financially to the care and rehabilitation of pets that are profoundly injured or ill. While we veterinarians do not advocate treating animals for selfish reasons, we do know that in many circumstances, badly broken bodies will heal if given proper care, love, and time. Such dedication extends far beyond any financial obligation or commitment, which can be sizable. The price these owners pay is in time and devotion, as much as in money. Often, these animals need round-the-clock attention to recover: Paralyzed animals must be turned over to prevent pressure sores, burned animals need their bandages changed frequently, some animals must be hand-fed. Such lengthy hospitalizations are costly, and often animals seem to be more comfortable and respond faster in their own home.

When a veterinarian dispenses a prescription or discharges a patient for follow-up care, either the doctor or a member of the hospital support staff takes the time to discuss the medicine or treatments with the owner. If the case is a complicated one and the choice has been made to have the owner participate by giving care at home, we painstakingly go over every aspect of their pet's nursing care, making sure that they understand exactly what to do and how they must perform each task for the safety and well-being of their animal. We explain the potential outcome to the best of our ability and discuss quality of life issues. Together, the family and the doctor decide how far we should take our care before their pet's quality-of-life is unsatisfactory.

This book is a manual of home-nursing care for the convalescing cat. I have found through experience that many explanations would be better understood if pet owners had diagrams to follow and written instructions to refer to once they got home. I chose to limit this book for both personal and practical reasons. Cats are admittedly my favorite animal to doctor, although I am the mistress not only to three cats but also a dog, Molly. From the practical standpoint, there are many approaches to the care and management of injured and sick cats that do not apply to dogs, and vice versa. So dogs will be dealt with another time.

If your cat has been to your veterinarian for illness or injury, chances are he or she may require some continuing treatment at home, whether it be medication, long-term "bed-rest" such as cage confinement for fractures, hand-feeding, or fluid administration. As I've already said, your participation in the convalescent care is very important. Once your veterinarian has examined your cat, made a diagnosis and recommendations for treatment, it's up to you to follow those instructions as carefully as possible to insure a speedy and complete recovery.

You may be one of those special people who has committed themselves to their cat through a long-term recovery from injuries or chronic illness. Perhaps long-term hospitalization is impractical or too expensive or you think your older and more sensitive cat may eat better and recover faster at home. With confidence and some instruction, you can play an important role in your pet's health care. This book is not meant to be a substitute for examination and primary care from your veterinarian. It is not a manual of diagnosis and treatment. You will learn the rationale for therapy and find simple written instructions and illustrations for common procedures that your veterinarian has already instructed you to do: medicating, applying compresses to wounds, etc. It also contains information on simple record-keeping, possible post-surgical problems, maintaining a bed or cage for a sick cat, and other useful techniques.

The third part of the book concerns cat diseases. Diseases are discussed in an encyclopedic approach. You'll see that clinical signs or symptoms can be the same for problems in different body systems. Part One talks about choosing a veterinarian and about what happens when your cat is admitted to the hospital. There is a glossary that demystifies commonly used medical terms and diagnostic tests.

When writing a book about animals, an author is always faced with a dilemma on how to handle the references to gender within the text. No one knows better than a veterinarian how irked people become when their pet is referred to by the incorrect sex. (I admit that I bristle too when somebody refers to my she-cat Willie as a he!) And we don't want to slight anyone by favoring one gender over another. So for the purposes of this book, I've tried to be consistent and have used the "he" and "she" gender reference in alternating chapters.

Lastly, a word of encouragement. Cats have a remarkable capacity to mend and heal, owing to their patience, adaptive natures, small, lightweight body frames, tolerance of bandages and other appliances, and receptiveness to human touch. Communicate closely with your veterinarian; together you make quite a team.

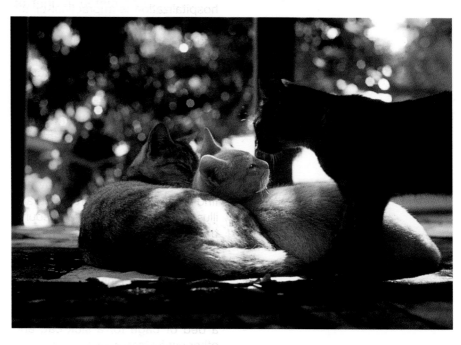

Acknowledgments

I am very grateful to the many friends and colleagues who have contributed to the production of this book. My thanks go to Don Reis and the editorial staff at Barron's Educational Series, Inc. for their guidance and dedication to their superior standards in education; Dr. Jean Lasser, Brenda Alexander, Amee Card, Janet Henderson, Sandy Brower, and Carly from Goodfriends Veterinary Clinic, Dr. Todd Minor, Peggy Dunn, Zinny and Bushy from the Groton-Ledyard Veterinary Hospital, and the Greater Nashua Humane Society, Nashua, New Hampshire for their generous cooperation in obtaining the photographs as well as their devotion to the welfare of animals, and excellence in veterinary medicine.

I am very pleased to acknowledge the work of photojournalists Don Himsel for coordinating and so professionally executing the photographs and Tami Plyler-Himsel for contributing the striking feature of the firefighter's rescue. That this book is rightfully a family affair makes the work ever more meaningful.

I am honored to thank Dr. Fredric Frye for his thoughtful review of the manuscript and continued encouragement. The time and effort given by the distinguished Dr. Frye is especially appreciated in light of his rigorous schedule. I extend my thanks to Dr. Barry Rathfon for teaching me to always do a thorough physical examination and to look inside every ear and every eye, every time. And lastly, a very special thanks to my husband, Richard, whose devotion to me and support for my work is proudly displayed on his license plate as: OH MEOW.

Carol Himsel Daly, D.V.M.
Winter 1994

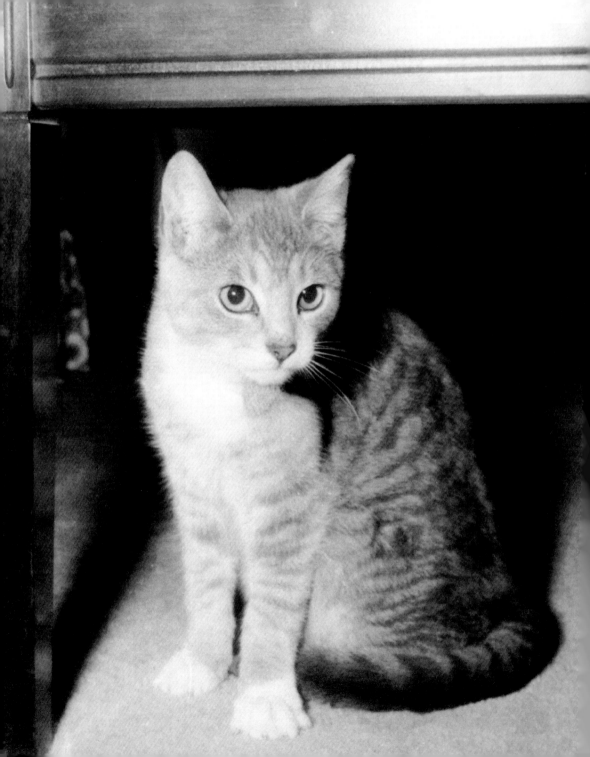

Chapter 1
Choosing a Veterinarian

WANTED

Person needed to care for important family members and members of the community. Minimum eight years post-secondary school training in anatomy, physiology, pathology, microbiology, parasitology, epidemiology, internal medicine, surgery, orthopedics, obstetrics, nutrition, pediatrics, gerontology, animal behavior (including human), for all domestic animals and birds. Aquatic medicine a plus. Master's degree in small business administration helpful. Must be available days, nights, weekends, and holidays.

Every pet owner has needs that are unique to his or her own circumstances, household, philosophy or attitudes about the role of pets. Consequently, veterinarians will wear many hats over the course of their professional lifetime in order to fulfill the needs of different pets and pet owners. Here are some factors to consider when you are looking for a veterinarian to care for your cat. Since each factor can add value to the relationship you establish, weigh the importance of each one carefully.

One Doctor or Two?

Or three, or four.... Historically, veterinary practices have been largely one-doctor facilities employing one or more assistants to perform receptionist and nursing duties. As veterinary medicine has become more sophisticated and specialized, veterinarians have moved toward working in teams in order to offer more services and better medicine. Large group practices are now very common. There are advantages to using group practices for veterinary

1

care. Because several veterinarians are working together, they can more easily afford state-of-the-art diagnostic equipment like fiberoptic endoscopes and ultrasound machines. Group practices often have doctors on staff with knowledge and possibly board certification in a specialty such as surgery or ophthalmology. Larger practices try to have staff clinicians with a broad range of special interests such as exotic or nondomesticated animal medicine for their clients with unusual pet birds or reptiles. Multi-doctor practices often provide their own 24-hour emergency service since the on-call responsibility can be shared. They may even staff the hospital for the entire 24-hour period. Because there are several doctors, it may be easier to get an appointment on short notice or on any day of the week.

On the other hand, you can lose the personalized attention of a single- or two-doctor practice in large practices. Solo practices offer security: You know the doctor, who in turn knows your cat, and you will never have to wonder, "Which doctor will I be seeing today?" Add to that a friendly, caring receptionist who has "been there forever," and the solo practice can seem very appealing. A busy and hectic multi-doctor hospital may not matter to you when you come in once a year for preventive care, but how comfortable would you be if your cat was seriously ill?

Also, don't assume that just because a practice or hospital has only one or two doctors, its equipment or medicine is second rate. Within the walls of every veterinary hospital are thousands of dollars invested in the same supplies and equipment found in human hospitals. And if a hospital chooses not to purchase and maintain its own ultrasound unit, for example, there are mobile veterinarians with ultrasound equipment who travel into hospitals to provide this service.

Cost Versus Value for Services

Cost for services is one of the most important considerations people must face when deciding on which veterinary hospital to use. Clients "shopping" for prices for examinations and vaccinations call daily. If you choose to do this, make sure that the receptionist or technician gives you a breakdown of what the fees represent.

Here's an example. A concerned cat owner calls Dr. Manx's office and asks, "How much does it cost to have my cat neutered?" The receptionist says, "Twenty-five dollars."

Next, the cat owner calls Dr. Birman's office and asks the same question. Here the receptionist responds by first asking, "What is your cat's name, and how old is he?" After you reply, the receptionist says, Dr. Birman charges fifty-five dollars. This fee includes an examination to make sure Binky is healthy and has no obvious problems that would put him at a greater risk for anesthesia. It also includes the anesthesia, and one night of hospitalization. Binky would come in to see us between 8 and 9 AM the morning of his surgery. He would go home after 9 AM the next day. Dr. Birman or our technician Joanie will call you after the operation, to let you know how everything went. To protect Binky and our other patients in the hospital from contagious diseases, he would need to be vaccinated prior to surgery. Do you have any other questions?"

Which hospital do you think that client is likely to trust with her cat? Dr. Manx's fees are lower, but which hospital offers more value? Actually, you don't know from the information given, but that's my point. Dollar price quotes alone rarely give you enough information about the care and consideration that goes into the services provided. *The care and consideration along with the quality of products and services (which includes the expertise of the doctors), equals the total value provided.*

Unfortunately, the caveat, "You get what you pay for," may apply to veterinary care, too. The low price may prove very disappointing. Suppose the client made an appointment and brought Binky to Dr. Birman's for vaccinations prior to the operation. While in the exam-

ination room, Joanie asked her some questions and learned that she was worried about fleas in the coming summer months. Joanie thoroughly explained the steps needed to protect Binky from fleas. She also recommended what to feed Binky after surgery. Finally, when she learned that the client was planning a vacation in August and needed a place to board her cat, Joanie gave the owner a brochure that outlined the boarding services provided by the hospital.

Can you see the value provided by this hospital? The staff probably saved this owner considerable expense and emotional concern down the road. No flea problem, no worry about Binky on vacation. Look for this kind of value when you compare costs.

And now a word about fees. Fees for services are set based on the expenses necessary to operate a veterinary hospital. These include mortgage and taxes, or rent on the building and land; insurance; salaries and benefits to employees; equipment purchases and maintenance; variable expenses like heat, electricity, and telephone bills; drugs and supplies; fees for licensing; continuing education; disposal of medical wastes; etc. After all that, the doctor pays himself or herself a salary. Third-party payments (health insurance) in veterinary medicine are not readily available or cost effective at this time. All those expenses must be met by fees collected for services. It would be lovely if health care for animals were available for nothing. Reality dictates otherwise.

A Warm and Caring Staff

No matter what your personal circumstances, goals, or priorities may be, you want to bring your cat to a veterinary hospital that has a warm and caring staff. And you may be thinking that because a person loves animals and works with them all day long, they will be warm and caring. Not true. I have been in several hundred animal hospitals and it is just amazing what some clients will put up with when it comes to the veterinary staff.

How do most clients evaluate the quality of the veterinary care available at any hospital? Most clients base this appraisal not on medical considerations, but rather on non-medical ones: the attitude of the receptionists, the cleanliness of the waiting room, the time it takes to get an appointment, and so forth. The qualifications of the doctors play much a lesser role—at least in the beginning.

One fact that has turned up in many surveys is that most clients stop going to a veterinary practice because they believe the staff does not care about their pet—*not because of dissatisfaction with the medical care or its cost.* And less than 5 percent of dissatisfied clients tell the doctor or the staff that they are unhappy. That means that a good doctor with a bad receptionist may never be aware of any problem. It also means that a client who loves the doctor but can't abide the staff may end up in another veterinary hospital.

Although a veterinary hospital's reason for being is to provide care for animals, this is only a small portion of our responsibility. Because animals cannot telephone for an appointment, drive to the office, describe their symptoms and write out a check, veterinary medicine is largely a "people profession." The best veterinary hospitals provide outstanding medical care by highly trained doctors and ancillary staff. They are also committed to "delight the customer"—you.

Hospital Hours

Most veterinary hospitals have a receptionist on staff to answer the telephone and a technician on duty to begin morning treatments by 8:00 AM, with doctor's appointments starting at the same time or shortly thereafter. Depending upon your own schedule and responsibilities, you may need to find a veterinary hospital that offers doctor's appointments early in the morning or later in the evening one or more days a week. Also inquire as to whether or not the doctor permits patients to be dropped off outside of regular doctor's hours, as long as the pet owner is accessible by telephone. Larger group practices are more likely to offer doctor's appointments on Saturdays too.

Most veterinary hospitals do not have a staff member within the building 24 hours a day. Many people are surprised to learn this. Usually, a staff member (assistant or doctor) checks on the animals and does treatments late in the evening. Afterwards, the animals are alone until a doctor or assistant comes in early in the morning. If a critical patient requires round-the-clock monitoring, one of several things happens. Sometimes a staff member stays at the hospital overnight. Sometimes the patient is transferred to an emergency clinic and comes back to the same hospital in the morning. Sometimes the patient (and the case) is sent to a referral hospital that does have a 24-hour staff. Ask your potential veterinarian which procedure is used at the hospital.

Emergency Services

Since animals don't always get sick during normal business hours, there may be times when you will need medical assistance in the evening, on weekends, or on holidays. There are a variety of ways that a veterinarian can provide that assistance. In rare cases, some practices have a staff clinician physically in the building and on call twenty-four hours a day. This, of course, is the best possible option, but it is a costly service for the hospital, so only the larger group practices or university teaching hospitals are likely to offer this.

To get around this dilemma, another option is to refer all after-hours calls to an emergency clinic in the area. Some emergency clinics are managed and staffed by doctors and technicians in the evening, and on weekends and holidays; they are specifically hired to work at this clinic by a group of veterinarians who support the clinic. Some groups of doctors will get together and take turns handling each other's emergency calls on a rotating basis. In this case, there is a chance that you may actually end up seeing your regular veterinarian.

If you want to be able to see your regular veterinarian for emergencies, you need to find one who takes his or her own calls. When you call the hospital after hours, you may speak to an answering service who contacts the doctor for you. Some veterinary hospitals have an answering machine that activates a pager when you leave a message. Either way, it will take some time for the doctor to return your call. Remember they're probably not sitting at home waiting for the phone to ring. They may be at the grocery store or a Little League game with their child, and will need to find a telephone.

Quality of Care

Think for a moment about the most famous and respected human hospitals that you know. The Mayo Clinic in Minnesota, the Memorial Sloan-Kettering Cancer Center in New York, or St. Jude's Children's Hospital in Texas might be on that list. These hospitals pioneer medical science and have extraordinarily sophisticated equipment and staff. Is this kind of hospital necessary for everyone, even people with serious illnesses? No, of course not. Chances are there is a fine medical center not too far away that has excellent doctors and nurses and state-of-the-art equipment. Hopefully, if you were to need what one of these famous hospitals had to offer, you could travel there and take advantage of it.

The same holds true for veterinary medicine. There are 27 veterinary schools (see Appendix) with teaching hospitals throughout the United States. The professors of clinical medicine and surgery are advanced-trained and board certified in virtually the same specialties—such as oncology and dermatology—as their human colleagues. There are also private referral practices in most states. These hospitals may or may not accept patients from the community. They do evaluate and treat patients sent to them by other veterinarians because of their expertise and facilities.

Just like people, most cats do not require the services of these hospitals. Excellent medical care can be found close by. Unless you have a medical background yourself, it can be difficult to evaluate the quality of medical care given at any one hospital. Here are some superficial things to look for that can give you some insight into the quality of care.

Certainly the physical characteristics of the facility are important. Examine the waiting room, parking lot and yard for cleanliness and odor. Are the magazines in the waiting room current? What kind of merchandising does the hospital do? Are the posters or bulletin boards informational for the season, or are they ripped, faded, or quote twenty-year-old statistics on disease incidence? These characteristics are important because they reflect the concern that the staff has in making their clients comfortable—to feel like guests. It also indicates the staff's interest in educating their clients on important animal health issues.

Let's move on to the staff itself. Do they dress professionally in clean attire? Does the receptionist answer the telephone by introducing herself and does she ask to help you before clicking you on hold? You have the right to have all your questions answered in a thorough and courteous manner. Remember, the staff is there to help you, not vice versa. A lousy receptionist is abrupt and gives as brief an answer as possible. She shows little pride in the hospital. A good receptionist smiles and is patient. A great receptionist smiles and is patient, even if there are three screaming children using the waiting room for a runway. Which receptionist would you want to encounter if your cat were hit by a car?

Most veterinarians are very proud of their facility and will happily give you a tour when time permits. That will give you an opportunity to examine the treatment areas and wards. Look inside the cages to see if the patients have something to lie on, and if the cages and runs are clean and dry. Use some judgment here, but don't hesitate to ask questions about kennel procedures. There may be some specific reason for a cage to be set up a certain way. For example, you may be concerned that an animal doesn't have a water bowl. This animal could be scheduled for surgery or may be undergoing a diagnostic procedure that requires that water be withheld.

You should learn how the hospital performs certain diagnostic procedures like laboratory analysis, electrocardiograms (EKG's), radiographs (x-rays), ultrasound, endoscopy, anesthesia, orthopedic

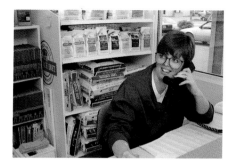

A good veterinary receptionist conveys information carefully and accurately to both the pet owner and the hospital staff.

surgery, etc. Larger hospitals have more equipment in-house. That doesn't mean that if some procedures like an EKG, for instance, can't be done right there, the hospital is substandard. The key point to establish is that the doctors do have access to these diagnostic tools or specialty services either through teaching hospitals, referral centers, a central hospital if this is a satellite facility, or "traveling" veterinarians, and that they are willing to use them or make the referral when necessary. Your cat may never need an ultrasound exam, but isn't it nice to know he could get one!

Although these recommendations refer back to the use of nonmedical factors to make important medical decisions, keep in mind that how you are treated and how your questions are answered does reflect on the quality of care at this hospital. You probably used the same criteria to chose a family doctor: How nice is the office, how friendly and professional is the staff, what are the office hours, who handles emergencies, what hospital affiliation do the doctors have, and how eager was everyone to satisfy my inquiries?

Credentials

State laws require that veterinarians post their license to practice medicine somewhere visible in the office. A license to practice certifies that they have graduated from an accredited school of veterinary medicine and have passed the national and state examinations to practice. Graduates of foreign schools go through an extremely rigorous process that includes testing and a year of clinical experience at an approved U.S. facility before being allowed to sit for the national and state examinations to obtain a license. Check the office for a license.

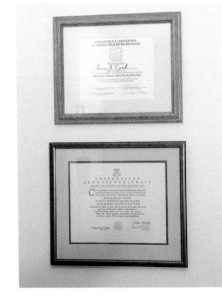

Veterinary technicians are the skilled equivalent of nurses in the human medical field.

Advanced training in a medical specialty such as surgery or radiology is obtained through an internship and residency program. Internships and residencies are not required by law. After completing these programs, a veterinarian applies for board certification to the specialty college. He or she must fulfill additional academic requirements such as publishing papers in medical journals, and sitting for examination before the board. If they pass—and it's tough—they become diplomates of the college for their specialty. Professional ethics requires that a doctor be a diplomate and board-certified in order to promote himself or herself as a "specialist" in any field. However, there are many excellent veterinarians with advanced training in areas of "special interest" who have not gone through a formal board certification process. (Note the difference here.)

Because of their expertise, board-certified veterinarians see animals that are referred by other veterinarians. Having a board certified veterinarian on staff means that the hospital can offer some services for which your cat would otherwise have to go to another hospital. (See Appendix for a list of some board certification specialties.)

All states define and regulate the types of procedures that technicians are allowed to do with and without supervision by a veterinarian. Some states also offer licensing.

Technicians who go through this process are called "registered," "certified," or "licensed" animal health technicians (R.A.H.T, C.A.H.T, or L.A.H.T.). Certification is obtained through examination. Most technicians receive on-the-job training, but there is "formal" training available through veterinary technician schools and programs at colleges and veterinary schools.

A technician does not have to have "formal" training to sit for the examination. Certified technicians may or may not be more qualified than noncertified technicians. Unfortunately, at this point in the professional licensure of technicians, the training and standards required by the doctors at the hospital is a better judge of skill than the certificate on the wall.

Special Medical Services

This would include the services given by board certified veterinarians that we have already discussed. Other special services to look for are house calls and home nursing assistance.

Nonmedical Services

When you travel for your work or for leisure, who looks after your cat? A friend or neighbor could check in if you are gone only a day or two, but what about longer absences? Now you need the services of a boarding facility. Many veterinarians offer boarding. They may board both dogs and cats, only cats, anyone's pets, or just their clients' pets. Even those with a no-boarding policy often make an exception for some clients, especially those with very old or very young pets or pets with chronic diseases like diabetes. If your veterinarian cannot board cats, ask if they can recommend a particular kennel or cattery in your area. They might have a special relationship with someone whom they know observes the boarders carefully and calls right away with any problems.

In recent years, we have seen an increase in the number of animal-care providers who visit your home so that your pets can stay in their own environment while you are away. This situation is ideal for cats. Chances are the staff at your veterinary hospital knows someone who has this kind of business or may even provide this service themselves. Again, your veterinarian may already have a close working relationship with someone whom he or she trusts to give medication or report any problems to the hospital immediately.

Other nonmedical services to consider are grooming, transportation or ambulance service, home delivery of prescriptions, products, or pet foods, behavior counseling and training (although this is mostly applicable to our canine companions), and private cremation.

Visiting Policy

Most veterinary hospitals permit pet owners to visit their pets during a long hospitalization. Some doctors encourage this practice, others only consent to this if requested. Even a generous open-door policy limits visits to certain hours set aside outside of the time for office calls and surgery, when the staff and doctors are extremely busy. Be sure to inquire about those hours and whether or not you must call ahead before stopping by.

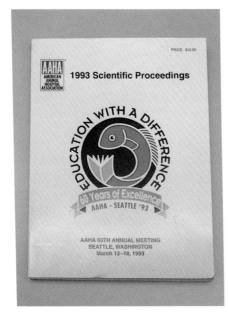

PRICE: $42.00

1993 Scientific Proceedings

EDUCATION WITH A DIFFERENCE

60 Years of Excellence
AAHA - SEATTLE '93

AAHA 60TH ANNUAL MEETING
SEATTLE, WASHINGTON
March 13–18, 1993

The American Animal Hospital Association sets voluntary standards for accreditation.

Certification

Depending upon the state where you live, your state Board of Veterinary Medical Examiners may do inspections of veterinary hospitals to see that they meet specific standards. These inspections may be voluntary or mandatory. The standards can vary from standards for practicing veterinary medicine all the way to physical upkeep. If you wish to inquire about any inspection requirements, contact your state board.

Nationally, there is an association called the American Animal Hospital Association (AAHA) that hospitals can join voluntarily. Hospitals achieve one to four years accreditation based on the level of excellence for hospital standards. The standards are determined by an AAHA committee and apply to all aspects of delivery of patient care, from the medical record to cleanliness of the facility. Accreditation requires on-site evaluation. It costs money to join this organization and to participate in the evaluation process, which is an ongoing process. AAHA also sponsors a national meeting for veterinarians yearly. You don't have to be an AAHA member to attend. The quality of speakers and continuing education at these meetings are some of the best.

There are a number of excellent hospitals that, for any number of reasons, are not AAHA members.

Just because a hospital is AAHA accredited, there is no guarantee that this is the best hospital in town. However, in my experience, if I were to move to a town and need a veterinarian, I would check out an AAHA member first. While it is no guarantee, it is the only independent, national "watchdog" (okay, maybe "watchcat" would be better) that is available. A directory of the national AAHA membership is published annually. If you are moving, your current veterinarian can tell you where the closest AAHA hospital is to your new home.

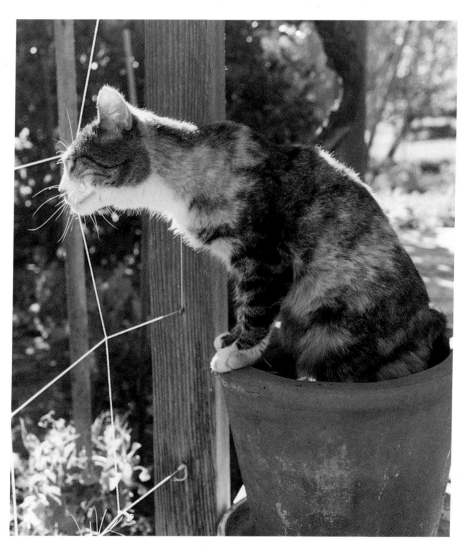

Chapter 2

What Happens When Your Cat Is Admitted to the Hospital

Admissions Process and Credit

Here comes Binky, back for his surgery. What can his owner expect? Since the cost of the neutering was an important consideration for her, the hospital has probably already given her an itemized estimate of expenses. This may or may not be routine for the veterinary hospital of your choice; some hospitals only give a written estimate if the pet owner asks for one. Written estimates are exactly that, an estimate. Should Binky experience problems with anesthesia or complications from the surgery, there may be additional charges.

Along with an estimate, Binky's owner will sign a hospitalization agreement. This agreement states what procedures will be performed and that his owner is giving her consent to have them done. It is a sort of contract. The signing of a hospitalization agreement is the same procedure a person would follow if admitted into a human hospital. In an emergency situation, a veterinary hospital may forego the formality of signing an agreement in the interest of saving time and the patient's life. Doctors usually don't go to the trouble of having an additional agreement signed every time another procedure or treatment is elected during a long or serious disease. Verbal agreements are made after a discussion with the pet owner on the best course of action.

After all the paperwork is completed, Binky's owner will ask a few last-minute questions about when his surgery will be done and when he can go home. If there is any question in her mind about the hospital payment policy, this is the time to ask. Most doctors, regardless of the species of animal or body part that they work on, require payment at the time the service is given. If the animal has medical insurance coverage, the pet owner then bills the insurance company for reimbursement. Bank cards are taken for convenience. Rarely do doctors bill on a regular basis. If you need the privilege of an account, make arrangements in advance of services. This is especially important in a catastrophic situation. All veterinarians have heard the words, "Do anything you can, Doc, never mind the cost," only to present a bill to a shocked pet owner two days later. The bill can be particularly devastating if the patient dies. A lot of people are hesitant to talk about charges and payments because they're afraid that someone will perceive them to be cold and heartless by bringing up the topic of cost up front. Don't be embarrassed! Because pet insurance isn't the ready safety net it is for people, the cost for services must be discussed right at the beginning, since the full payment is going to come directly out of the owner's pocket. Veterinarians are very accustomed to discussing the economics of a case and are willing to work with a pet owner in catastrophic situations. That doesn't mean doing the work for free, but it does mean extending some sort of credit in good faith if bank cards are not an option.

Accommodations for the Patient

If you've had an opportunity to tour your veterinary hospital, you're probably already familiar with the kennel procedures. Binky will be placed in a cage labeled with a card marked with information about him and his owner. Some veterinary hospitals also put identifying neck bands on the patients just as human hospitals use wrist bands. Patients that are scheduled for surgery that day do not get food or water. Once Binky is sufficiently recovered from anesthesia, he will be given water and a litterbox. If your cat and child are closely bonded, it might be a good idea to have the child bring your cat into the ward and stay while the assistant gets him settled in. A few adults could benefit from this, too. Even I get a little emotional when I have to leave my pets in the hospital!

In one hospital in California where I practiced for many years, our veterinary technician Chirp had the self-appointed task of providing what I liked to call Cage Karma. Using small, empty boxes lined with fleece pads and towels, Chirp created dark and quiet labyrinths for the cats, or draped the front of the cages with cloth or paper to dim the noise and lights. She suspended empty syringe cases with a string as batting toys for the kittens. We had a collection of stuffed animals that clipped onto the cage bars or got tucked into a corner for company. Chirp made the patients feel better because she gave them solitude and a place to escape from the noise and commotion of the hospital. Less stress can mean faster recovery.

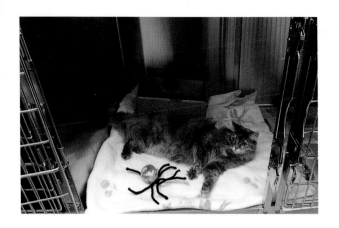

Visitation and Discharge

If your cat will be hospitalized or boarded for several days, you might ask about bringing in a favorite toy or blanket for a bed. Sometimes I think the cat appreciates having a little something from home, other times I'm not so sure. I do know that it does a cat owner a world of good, so I encourage this with a warning that something may go in the laundry and not be recovered when it's time to go home.

Like most hospital stays, Binky will be away from home for only a day or two. Should he be there longer, his owner might want to visit. Ask the staff about the hospital's visiting policy. Your visit could be very helpful for the staff if you could assist in feeding. Your visit could also be timed with dressing changes or other nursing procedures and be a good consultation time between you and the doctor.

Many cat owners ask about exercise and socialization while their friend is in the hospital. Certainly if the cat is ill, he won't want much in the way of company and playtime. For those patients recovered enough to get out and stretch their legs, many hospitals let the cats out to roam the ward as their cages are cleaned. Some hospitals have set aside playrooms for this purpose. We used to bring the noninfectious patients into the doctors' office where they'd sit on our desks and assist with the paperwork. To what degree your cat will be given one-on-one attention and socialization will depend on the facility and available time. If this is an important consideration for you, ask the hospital staff.

Chapter 3
Preventive Care

Although the number of households with cats is now greater than the number of households with dogs, less than half of those cats receive regular veterinary preventive care. Popular opinion has placed a lesser value on the life of a cat than on a dog, whose companionship is a bit more obvious to some. Why spend any money on it when you can "just get another cat"? And even if a pet owner loves his or her cat, many are ignorant of even the minimal steps that could be taken to control preventable diseases, let alone the advanced medical services that are available. All this is true, despite the high profile cats have in our society through the millions of dollars spent on cat-food advertising, cat magazines, cat shows, and stores devoted to the plethora of cat paraphernalia.

Presumably if you're reading this book, you're already aware of the need for preventive health care for your cat. This should serve as a reminder as to why you take the steps you do and as a reference so you can educate others about important cat health issues.

Vaccinations

When a kitten is born, it does not have an active immune system with which to fight infection. This leaves the kitten vulnerable to diseases that adult cats would take in stride. When a kitten nurses for the first time, he receives immune protection from his mother in the form of antibodies, present in the first milk or colostrum. This type of immunity is called passive immunization. The antibodies in colostrum are rapidly absorbed into the kitten's bloodstream and distributed throughout the body. The absorption of antibodies can take place for only a few short hours after birth. After that

Kittens absorb protective antibodies in the colostrum or "first milk" during the first 24 hours of life.

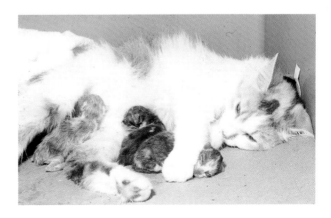

time, additional colostrum will do no good; the antibodies are simply digested along with everything else and cannot be absorbed. That's why it's so important that newborns begin to nurse as soon as possible after birth or Caesarean section, so that they can absorb as much of the colostral antibodies as possible during that brief window of opportunity.

Once the antibodies are circulating inside the kitten's system, they go about the business of fighting off germs. Antibodies don't last forever though, especially those that are transferred from the mother. These antibodies are depleted or used up through attrition, so that over several weeks the amount of mother's antibodies declines to insignificant and ineffective amounts.

As the mother's antibodies are depleted, the kitten's own immune system is taking shape. At about eight weeks of age, the kitten's immune system is sufficiently ready to be challenged by the first inoculation against the common respiratory viruses of cats. Because the residual antibodies from the mother will interfere with the development of a strong response to that vaccine, kittens should be given boosters every three to four weeks until they are 16 weeks of age. It is impossible to predict just when the mother's antibodies are sufficiently used up, and when the kitten's immune system will respond appropriately to the vaccine. So, a series

of boosters is necessary in order to insure that the kitten's immune system has been stimulated to produce adequate amounts of its own protective antibodies.

What about adult cats? Unlike kittens, healthy adolescent and adult cats are fully capable of responding to a vaccine the first time it is given. If the initial kittenhood vaccinations have been delayed until after four months of age, these cats should receive two inoculations, approximately three to four weeks apart, against most of the common cat diseases. The same rule of thumb should be applied to adult stray cats whose vaccination status is, of course, unknown. The first inoculation will stimulate an immune response. The second inoculation imparts a stronger and more long-lasting response, a sort of memory to the system. Keep in mind that although older cats do not have to worry about maternal antibodies interfering with the first inoculation, one inoculation is not sufficient to produce adequate protection. They must have the second one that results in the long-lasting effect.

After the initial series of vaccinations, cats should receive booster shots once a year in order to keep the memory of that immunity strong. Consider that, on the average, a cat can live about 15 or 16 years, while its owner may live 75 years. One year may represent not quite 10 percent of a cat's lifespan.

But 10 percent of the owner's lifetime is about 7 years! Annual vaccinations against the respiratory diseases for your cat would be similar to your receiving a flu vaccine every seven years throughout your own lifetime. Given the volatile nature of human flu virus, this would be highly ineffective in protecting you! Luckily, cat viruses are a lot more stable, and annual vaccinations are usually adequate to protect them, unless the cat is severely stressed.

Which leads us to consider the need for vaccinations in geriatric cats. One might assume that after all those years of boosters, that once a cat were to reach a ripe old age, vaccinations would no longer be necessary. On the contrary, as the cat ages, so does the immune system. The immune response can wane, leaving the older cat vulnerable once again. Annual vaccinations keep the immune response strong, and are an important part of geriatric care.

So why would some cats become sick with these diseases even after vaccination? The answer to that question can be obvious or speculative. First of all, the cat may not have received an adequate number of boosters, or there may have been a large amount of maternal antibodies to interfere with the inoculation series. No vaccine will protect 100 percent of the time. A cat can come in contact with a particularly powerful or virulent strain of a virus that overwhelms the immune system. Or the immune system can be diminished due to stress associated with boarding, moving, inclement weather, new members of the household, poor nutrition, immunosuppressive viruses, or other underlying diseases. Compared to unvaccinated cats, cats that have been properly vaccinated will develop only a mild form of the disease during a "vaccine break." Some cats will carry a virus in their body, undetected and without causing disease, until some stress lowers their resistance. Vaccinations may be ineffective in these cats.

Table 1 lists the common diseases against which cats are vaccinated. Your veterinarian will recommend all or some of these vaccines, depending upon your cat's risks of contracting one of them in your area. Even if your cat is of the totally indoor variety, he should be properly vaccinated against feline viral rhinotracheitis, calicivirus, and panleukopenia, which are highly contagious, and rabies, which is highly fatal.

Serologic Testing

Most veterinarians recommend routine serologic testing of all kittens and newly acquired adult cats for feline leukemia virus infection. A general definition of serologic testing is given in the Glossary (see page 171) along with a discussion

Table 1
Common cat diseases and their vaccines

Vaccine	Initial	Maintenance
Panleukopenia	2 doses, 4 weeks apart beginning at 8 weeks of age.	Annually. Special vaccine required for pregnant queens.
Calicivirus	Same as panleukopenia.	Annually.
Rhinotracheitis	Same as panleukopenia.	Annually.
Chlamydia	Same as panleukopenia.	Annually.
Feline infectious peritonitis	2 doses 4 weeks apart beginning at 16 weeks of age, in high risk catteries, households, and shelters where virus is endemic.	Annually.
Feline leukemia virus	2 or 3 doses, 4 weeks apart only after a negative FeLV test.	Annually.
Rabies	Dose at 3 months of age, then 1 year later.	According to local laws or manufacturer's recommendation. Precautionary after: 1) every wound of unknown origin; 2) every bite wound from animal with unknown vaccination history; 3) every bite from animal with lapsed vaccinations.

of the types and interpretation of feline leukemia virus testing. See page 124 for a discussion of this virus. Kittens and cats that test negative should be vaccinated. There has been a lot of debate within the veterinary and lay community surrounding this recommendation. First, none of the vaccines have been shown to be totally effective in producing the necessary immunities under laboratory testing, independent of the manufacturer. Secondly, some veterinarians do not feel that it is necessary to vaccinate cats that are never going to go outdoors.

Leukemia virus vaccines have improved tremendously since their introduction by a single manufacturer in the early 1980s. Although the laboratory evaluations have not proven them to be as effective as hoped, out in the real world under natural exposure situations, they do seem to afford substantial protection. The initial side effects, mostly pain on injection, have diminished too. My personal opinion is that since reasonably good protection is afforded, and because side effects are largely inconsequential, kittens and cats should be vaccinated. This applies to cats risking exposure. Remember that even if your cat stays totally indoors today, that may change at some time. Almost all boarding kennels and veterinary hospitals also require vaccination prior to admission to prevent accidental transmission through contact.

Serologic testing for feline immunodeficiency virus is becoming more routine. There is no vaccine available at this time; however, infection with this virus will affect the immune system and knowing the immune status of the cat may influence some decisions that you as an owner might make about this cat's lifestyle. You may choose to keep this cat indoors to lower the risk of injury and illness. And although the virus is only transmitted through bite wounds and not casual contact, you may choose not to have any other cats. We don't know a lot about the signifi-cance of infection with FIV; in other words, how the virus affects life-span. It is clear that many cats will live for years with the infection before it becomes a problem clinically, if ever.

Internal Parasite Control

A discussion of the life cycle and diseases caused by these parasites is included in Part II of this text. Kittens should have their feces examined for parasites twice, once at nine weeks of age and again about one month later. Thereafter, cats who spend any time outdoors should have a fecal examination yearly. Fecal parasite examinations are also a routine step in diagnosing the cause of vomiting and diarrhea in kittens or cats, so always provide your veterinarian with a fresh stool sample for analysis at the time of consultation for these problems.

Feces are examined for parasites in one of four ways. Direct observation will identify some tapeworms and heavy roundworm infections. Such cats or kittens may eliminate a number of mature adult worms in the feces (or vomitus). The direct smear technique is used to identify some protozoal parasites like *Giardia*. For this test, a swab of stool is applied to a glass slide with a drop of saline (salt water) and examined for organisms. The most common method of stool analysis for parasites is the fecal flotation test. The fourth method is called a Baerman analysis and is done to identify larvae from lungworm parasites. (See page 142.)

The treatment for internal parasites will depend upon the parasite itself, the age of the cat, and other existing conditions.

Neutering

At the time of this writing, there are no accurate statistics to tell us how many unwanted animals are euthanized each year. There just simply isn't a committee or group established to keep records from every shelter or animal-control facility. One estimate from the oldest and largest humane organization in the United States, the American Society for the Prevention of Cruelty to Animals in New York City, claims that 10,000,000 animals had to be destroyed in this country in 1991. Add to that figure the unknown number that died from disease, accidents, and starvation and what results is waste and suffering of tragic magnitude. In the PBS program "Throwaway Pets," Roger Caras, president of the ASPCA, tells us that if a single pair of cats mate and produce offspring, and all their offspring mate and produce more offspring and so forth, in seven years there would be 150,000 cats. Unless your cat is a show-quality purebred in both conformation and temperament, he or she should be neutered to prevent accidental pregnancy and unwanted kittens. The myth claiming that neutering causes cats and other animals to become fat and lazy is untrue. Too much food causes obesity. And "having one litter" will not make a cat more affectionate or a better pet. You will not be depriving him or her of any inborn "need" for procreation by neutering your cat. You won't be depriving them of anything at all.

Procedures for Males

Male cats are called "toms" until they are neutered and then they are called "premiers." It is to their credit that most associations recognize the premier class and allows these animals to show in competition. This is in contrast to the American Kennel Club which does not permit neutered dogs to compete. Cat owners can enjoy the excitement of cat shows and still have their cats neutered.

By convention, male cats are neutered at about eight months of age, or as I like to tell an owner, "the day before he starts to spray!" Some humane shelters will neuter a male as early as 12 weeks of age and for good reasons. The kittens recover very quickly from the surgery and seem to have less discomfort, although even older cats do not demonstrate much discomfort anyway. By neutering before adoption, the shelter does not have to worry about the adoptive owner complying with the standard agreement to have the kitten neutered at a later date. Some veterinarians do not like to neuter cats at such a young age because they believe that it will result in underdevelopment of the urethra and predispose the cat to urethral blockage common with feline lower urinary tract diseases. This theory has not been well-supported through research. Of course, if it's a big, beefy tomcat that you're after, you would have to wait a couple of years to neuter your male and allow him to breed and develop the characteristic broad head and jowls. Those physical characteristics don't regress after neutering.

Neutering your male cat usually involves castration. The scrotum is antiseptically prepared for surgery and an incision is made over the testicles. The testicles are removed from the scrotum and the blood supply and spermatic cords are tied. The incisions are not sutured. Despite this being a rather unsanitary area of the body, infection after this procedure is rare and recovery is rapid.

An alternative procedure to castration is vasectomy. For this procedure, the scrotum is also prepared antiseptically for surgery. An incision is made and the spermatic cords are identified, tied, and cut. The testicles remain in the scrotum and continue to produce testosterone. This cat will continue to perform all the objectionable male behavior: territorial urine spraying, roaming, fighting, and the arduous pursuit of females in heat.

Procedures for Females

Female cats are called "queens." Females are usually neutered at about six months of age, although again, some shelters will perform this surgery at 12 weeks. After six months of age, and occasionally earlier, females will begin to have "heat" or estrous cycles (see page 98). Because some cats will not exhibit any behavioral signs of estrus the first time around and yet be entirely capable of becoming pregnant, females should be confined indoors if possible, until they are neutered.

The neutering procedure for females is an ovariohysterectomy, not too surprisingly called in lay terms, "a spay." If you've had your cat neutered, she's been ovariohysterectomized, or "spayed." (That's pronounced: spaa-d, not spaad-ed.) And although you may have had a dozen cats spayed in your lifetime, and your veterinarian may have performed hundreds of these surgeries, this is far from an innocuous, minor procedure. It involves an incision that enters the abdominal cavity. The ovaries are identified and withdrawn through the incision. The blood vessels that nourish the ovaries come directly from the aorta, the largest artery in the body. The ovarian arteries must be securely tied off and severed.

Additional sutures are placed around the blood vessels that supply the Y-shaped uterus before both the uterus and the ovaries are removed. Then the incision is closed in several layers. Your cat may or may not have sutures in the skin layer that need to be removed at a later date.

This same procedure in women usually requires six to eight weeks for recovery. In contrast your cat will most likely begin to move around normally and have a normal appetite and habits as early as 24 hours after the surgery. Don't be fooled by this rapid return to normal. Confine your cat indoors and follow the instructions outlined in After Surgical and Dental Procedures, page 93.

Dental Care

For an explanation of one method for brushing your cat's teeth, see page 86. I recommend that you do this at least three times a week. At the time of your cat's annual physical examination and vaccinations, ask your veterinarian to evaluate your cat's teeth and assess the need for a thorough dental prophylaxis. Every cat's needs are unique; some, especially in the Siamese breed, can use a careful cleaning and polishing under the gum line every year. Other cats will need this only once or twice in their lifetime.

One word about scraping teeth. Some groomers offer this service, as do some veterinarians as a temporary measure until proper dentistry can be performed. Scraping teeth involves chipping off the large pieces of tartar with a sharp dental scaler while the cat is awake. This can improve the appearance of teeth cosmetically and can make it easier for some animals to eat. However, it also etches the enamel surface of the tooth, predisposing it to rapid return of the tartar.

The only proper method for cleaning teeth is to use a ultrasonic or rotary scaler like the ones your dentist would use on you. The teeth are cleaned on all surfaces and below the gums where cavities often occur in cats. After scaling, the teeth are polished to remove the surface etching. Some veterinarians also use a fluoride treatment to seal the teeth against cavities.

All this requires that your cat be put under anesthesia. A thorough examination for infection, cavities, and broken teeth, and proper cleaning and polishing cannot be accomplished while an animal is awake. Elderly cats are often the ones that need this type of dental work the most. To minimize the risks associated with anesthesia, your veterinarian will probably require pre-anesthetic laboratory evaluation of kidney and liver function. If there are other associated problems like a heart murmur, chest radiographs or x-rays and an EKG are advisable.

If all this seems rather elaborate and involved, consider what state your teeth and gums might be in if you went your whole life without brushing your own teeth and visiting a dentist. The health benefits obtained from routine preventive dental care are easier to understand if you have ever had a cat that acts reasonably "normal" despite the presence of fetid cat breath and bleeding gums. Once that cat's mouth is attended to and the infection is under control, you often see a personality change, with the cat becoming more affectionate and social. Eating habits also change. And this cat is at less of a risk for secondary effects of the chronic oral infection, like heart and kidney disease that can without question shorten his life.

Flea Control

To control fleas effectively, you must attack them at every part of the life cycle. To take the easy route and simply apply a flea collar or give a weekly bath will doom you to failure. Unless you live in a climate that does not support fleas, managing rather than eliminating a flea problem is the best you can do for your indoor-outdoor cat. Management can give you excellent results with only an occasional pest on your pet.

Effective flea control mandates that you use some insecticides. The so-called natural methods of flea control using herbs, garlic, nutritional yeast or other sources of B-vitamins, ultrasonic flea collars and boxes do not work, no matter how hard you wish that they would, even if it was your very best and trusted friend who swore by this method. All insecticides are not heinous and lethal. Some, such as the pyrethrins derived from a certain species of chrysanthemum, are natural botanicals, and are highly effective at killing fleas quickly. Your veterinarian can give you up-to-date information about flea control products.

Safety and effectiveness also depend upon the proper application and use of flea products. Manufacturers of these products have detailed instructions for entire flea control programs that include instructions for each step and product. Some programs have a toll-free telephone number for technical services. You can call and discuss your specific circumstances with a trained technician who will know more about the products you are using and how to get the most from the program. Some manufacturers even go so far as to offer a guarantee.

Insecticides are still the backbone of all flea programs, although they are losing ground to some newer and more effective approaches. They have a variable degree of three properties: to kill fleas on contact, to repel fleas, and to have residual action once they are applied to either the cat or the environment. Insecticides only kill adult fleas although some kill larvae. In recent years, researchers have developed a number of hormones called insect growth regulators that work only on fleas, not animals or the people that handle them. These hormones cause the eggs to dry up and not hatch. Where insecticides fail to kill eggs, these hormones essentially render the fleas sterile and break the flea life cycle. It is only by breaking this life cycle that fleas can be effectively controlled.

Before the development of insect hormones, boric acid powder was just about the only alternative to environmental insecticides available. Applied to the environment, boric acid powder reduces the humidity in the microenvironment (for example, the carpet) of the flea. Flea larvae just hate being in a low-humidity environment. Unfortunately, simply sprinkling boric acid powder around doesn't work very well. It must be manufactured and applied properly to be effective. There are a few boric acid-derivative flea control products for the environment that you can purchase and there are some professional flea control companies that specialize in this service. These are ideal for anyone who needs to avoid even the safest of environmental insecticides.

The Life Cycle of the Flea

Let's look at the flea life cycle. Of the fleas that parasitize dogs and cats, the adult fleas live their life on the animal. (For other flea species this is not so.) The adult female feeds by sucking blood, and mates and lays eggs on your cat. Blood is the sole food source for the adult flea, and because the female flea is laying enormous numbers of eggs, she is feeding frequently. The blood meal is digested and excreted as flea feces which looks like little specks of black pepper in your cat's coat. This is sometimes the only evidence that you find of a flea infestation. The flea eggs and feces fall off your cat. You can find this where your cat sleeps, and if the area is wet, the feces will dissolve and appear as blood specks. I have had more than one "emergency" with a cat brought in for bleeding from some unknown source when the owner found blood in the sink where the cat likes to sleep! You can try this for yourself. If your cat is scratching and yet you are having difficulty actually finding fleas, wet a paper towel and lay it out on a flat surface. Have your cat sit near the towel. Ruffle the fur at the base of the tail and around the neck so that any debris and loose hair falls onto the towel. Rub the specks that fall with your finger. Reddish-brown streaks appear as the flea feces become wet. This is dried blood from your cat.

The eggs hatch out tiny, translucent larvae that you can also see in areas where your cat spends time, if you look closely enough. The larvae feed mostly on the flea feces as well as skin scales and other organic debris. Flea larvae will not survive in dry climates with a relative humidity of less than 50 percent. But even in dry climates, deep between carpet fibers and shaded areas of the lawn and under bushes, there can be microenvironments that support the larvae.

Flea larvae spin a sticky cocoon and enter a pupa stage. This stage can last from a few days up to several months. If conditions are right, the pupae hatch and out comes a new adult flea seeking a host from which to suck a blood meal. This newly hatched adult must find another suitable host within three or four days or it will die. The pupae lie dormant if there is no host, such as the cat, for the next stage to feed on. For example, say you go on vacation for two weeks and your cat stays at the Cat Spa while you are gone. When the two of you return home, the pupae are stimulated to hatch by the vibrations of your footsteps and the carbon dioxide that you and your cat breathe off. Within a few days, the pupae have hatched and the new adults are covering your cat and your ankles.

Insecticides kill adult fleas. Some insecticides kill the larvae, too. If the adult fleas or the eggs have been treated with an insect growth regulator, the eggs are not viable and will not hatch. The weak link in the available technology for flea control is with the pupae. There is currently no chemical or hormone capable of killing the pupal stage. That's why a single environmental treatment is ineffective. Even if it were possible to kill off every adult, larvae, and egg, the pupae will survive to hatch out a new crop of adults.

A Program for Total Flea Control

Effective flea control involves treating the cat and the environment. While flea baths have a quick-kill effectiveness and can eliminate the adult fleas on your cat, flea baths have no residual effect. Once the soap is washed off, the newly hatched adults will jump right back on. Residual flea control on the cat means using an insecticidal spray, powder, dip or foam after the cat is bathed. This is also where flea collars fit in. They can help to keep the population of fleas down.

Flea combs have special teeth that trap the flea as it runs through the fur. It is possible to remove the fleas mechanically using a flea comb and thereby not use an insecticide on the cat. In households with a small flea-control problem, this approach may be feasible for removing most but probably not all of the adult fleas. Because fleas move between the hairshafts with ease and agility, and because the newly hatched adults are small, some fleas will escape the comb and go on to feed, lay eggs, and defecate dried blood.

Keep in mind that all the pets in the household must be involved in your flea-control program. Most people willingly go through all the necessary steps with the family dog. Let's face it, when it comes to baths and flea spray, Bowser is a lot more cooperative than Fluffy! But if you let even one member of your four-legged household slip by, even if you never see fleas on that particular elusive cat, that's the one that the fleas will be attracted to first. You may see very few to no fleas on that pet—he probably grooms them off fairly effectively. But be aware that before Fluffy has a chance to nab those fleas, they feed and lay eggs.

Environmental control means using insecticides and insect-growth regulators in areas where your cat spends most of his time: in the house and parts of the yard. Room foggers, aerosol or pump sprays should be used in your cat's favorite rooms, under and on the furniture where your cat sleeps, and along hallways where your cat walks. You may not need to apply these products to every room. For instance, if your cat is not allowed in an allergic person's bedroom, it is unlikely that there would be any flea eggs or larvae there. If you decide to use a flea comb to control adult fleas on the cat, you should still treat the environment with an insecticide that kills larvae and contains an insect growth regulator.

Likewise, it is also important to treat certain areas of your yard. This is an important reservoir for fleas often overlooked by owners. I'm not advocating that you spray the entire back forty acres, only those places where your cat likes to spend the most time. This would include places like under the rose bush where your cat crouches waiting to ambush your ankles as you stroll by, or in the cool dampness under the porch on a hot summer day.

Because the pupae are resistent to all chemicals, for your initial anti-flea campaign you should treat the environment twice, about three weeks apart. The first treatment should kill most of the adults, larvae, and eggs. The second treatment will kill the newly emerged adults. After the initial set of environmental treatments, you will need to maintain your control by periodically treating the environment, and regularly applying a spray, powder, or foam to your cat. Failure of any flea control program is usually due to use of ineffective products, incorrect application, inappropriate timing of applications, or failure to treat an area of the environment serving as a reservoir for flea eggs, larvae, and pupae.

Grooming

Although cats are fastidiously clean by nature, some cats need a little extra help. Grooming your cat provides several benefits. First, regular brushing and inspection will alert you early on to any skin problems, lumps, bumps, or fleas. It can help your cat to become accustomed to being handled. Brushing can be a pleasurable interaction between you and your pet that satisfies your cat's need for attention and can reduce anxiety and even blood pressure in people. By removing loose fur you help to reduce the incidence of hairballs and the amount of cat hair on the seat of your best friends' pants when they sit on your cat's favorite chair.

For routine brushing of short-haired cats, use a flat brush with short wire bristles called a slicker brush. This is the best tool I know to remove the loose undercoat and prevent matting. For long-haired breeds, a longer and softer bristled brush will de-tangle without breaking the hair-shaft. Small matts can be removed by just pulling with your fingers or with a matt comb. If your cat's fur has matted because of a heavy shed, it may be necessary to shave the matts out with a professional clipper. This is best done for you by a groomer. Be extremely cautious if you use scissors to cut matts out yourself. It is very easy to misinterpret just where the matt ends and where the cat's skin begins and end up lacerating your cat.

Aside from brushing, sometimes it will be necessary to give your cat a bath; see page 83. Always follow the label on the shampoo for lathering instructions unless your veterinarian advises otherwise.

Check your cat's paws for ingrown nails. This is especially important as they get older and may retain the old sheathes that will become embedded in the pads. Page 35 will instruct you on how to trim your cat's claws.

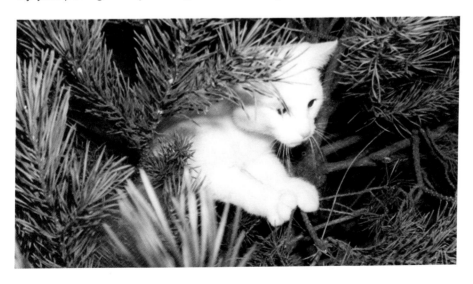

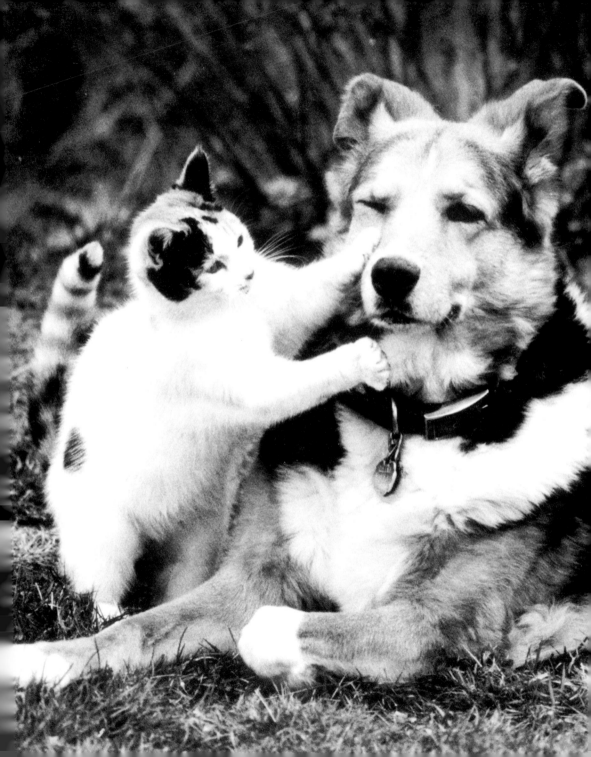

Chapter 4
Achieving Cooperation

The one trait for which cats are either loved or despised is their aloofness, the attitude of reserve and superiority over all other creatures that cats almost universally exhibit. Kittens are another matter, for they seem to look at life as one never-ending hunt, every movement as a potential prey, and other animals as amusements.

Sometime around five or six months of age, a kitten's view of the world changes, and it begins to be more selective about with whom it keeps company. My cat Cocoa is an uncommon exception; he sits on anyone's lap who will tolerate his drooling and kneading. Other cats will vanish, and I do mean vanish, at the first sign of a stranger. Most will observe us at a distance, judging the safety of the situation, our worthiness for their trust, and what possible benefit to them an interaction could bring. If we score high on all accounts we have a friend and see them ask with pleading eyes as they weave underfoot, "Do you

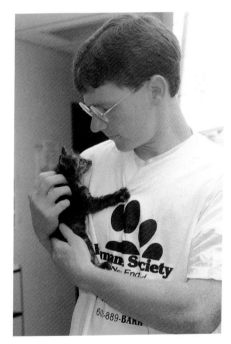

Humane Society workers and volunteers provide care and love to millions of unwanted animals each year. Support them by having your cat neutered.

know how to work the can opener?" With personalities in mind, anyone wishing to help a cat must first gain his or her cooperation. The method you use depends a lot on your relationship with the cat, the urgency of the situation, your

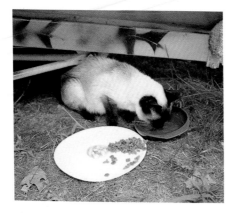

Leave food and water near a stray cat's safe haven.

All day long neighbors and friends tried to coax the kitty down from the pole, calling sweetly to it and leaving tasty offerings at the bottom. But no amount of comforting, no promise of food, no urging at all could persuade this cat to retreat. It stayed there all night, sometimes letting out a pathetic meow.

The next morning, one would-be hero decided that if food were dangled right in front of his face the cat would without a doubt inch his way down the pole. This fellow chose a piece of bologna as bait. He shimmied and struggled up the pole and approached the cat as closely as he could without touching the power lines and dangled his piece of bologna. The cat observed his benefactor with suspicion, judged his safety to be poor, and therefore unworthy of trust. The bologna was of no benefit whatsoever, and the cat decided to stay put. The man was forced to come down in defeat.

safety and his, and whether or not you have someone to help you. I once knew a cat that climbed up a high-tension power line pole, presumably after a bird. The bird flew away of course, leaving the cat perched about fifty feet in the air among the buzzing wires. The power line ran between a farmer's field and a very nice neighborhood. Not only did the owner of this cat discover its predicament as she glanced out her kitchen window, so did a number of the neighbors.

The very distraught owner of the cat began calling the power company and the fire department for assistance. She was met with a cold response. No one had a long enough ladder and besides, "Just leave that cat alone lady, and he'll come down on his own. Have you ever seen a cat carcass in a tree?"

When all else fails, call your veterinarian. The cat had been up this pole in the blazing 100° degree sun for nearly two days. Several logical and one very illogical approach to a

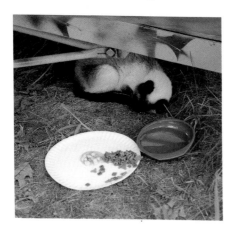

It takes some time to develop trust.

rescue had been tried. My approach was different; it was political. A second call to the power company revealed why no one would help. So many linemen had been mauled while attempting to rescue stranded cats that the company had changed its policy and would no longer respond to these calls. I related the story about the dangling bologna and pointed out how unfortunate it would be if someone were electrocuted trying an equally heroic measure, not to mention the publicity that would ensue if the owner called the local newspaper. Within an hour, an operator with a cherry picker and a cat carrier arrived. Up he went and, upon seeing the carrier, in went the cat. So you see, the bologna worked.

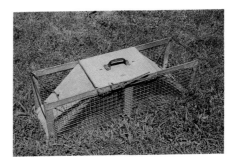

Feed and grain and hardware stores sell Have-A-Heart traps for removing unwanted wildlife and feral cats.

Food as a Motivator

Food is a primary motivator for most cats. Many injured strays have been coaxed into trusting by a square meal. Take your time. It could take several days or weeks of regular feeding before he trusts you enough to come into the house or allow you to pick him up. No injured or sick stray is worth the potential danger of a bad cat bite. If he's in really bad shape and you don't want to wait too long, you might be able to borrow a Have-A-Heart trap from a local humane organization. Consider the local laws pertaining

to rabies and feral dogs and cats before you get involved in rescuing any stray, especially if he is acting sick.

Food is probably a motivator for your own cat, too. If your veterinarian says it's all right for your convalescing cat to go out, time his treatments to mealtimes. Feed him something he really enjoys, and he'll arrive home with an uncanny precision.

Cats who live primarily outdoors, make irregular appearances at home, or belong to owners with restrictive work schedules should be confined indoors for the duration of their treatment. This isn't cruel; you're not going to make your cat neurotic by refusing to let him answer the call of the wild. It's more important that you provide proper and timely care to insure a rapid recovery and return to normal life.

Where to Work

Now that your cat's available and you actually have to do something to him, we need to talk about

Perform all procedures on a firm, non-slip, waist-level surface. The bed, couch, or floor are not appropriate.

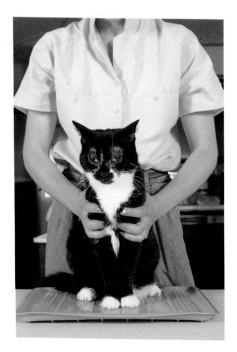

use the element of surprise to your advantage. Some people find it easier to work sitting cross-legged on the floor with their cat tucked in their lap.

Once on familiar territory, the average cat will sit or lie on his side for inspection, at least by its owner. Place him on the table facing away from you, so that he can't back up. Have an assistant scratch behind his ears or under his chin to draw attention away from what you want to look at or do.

If a cat chooses not to cooperate, the first thing he'll do is try and run away. Put a rubber kitchen sink liner on whatever surface you're working on to give him something to dig into with his claws. Don't use a bath towel; they slide around too much and lead the cat to panic. Gently but firmly, hold the cat on the table. A cat will definitely struggle to escape if three or four hands grab, squeeze, or squash him to the table.

Rather than either cooperate or run away, a few cats stand their ground. A cat first uses its posture, voice, front claws, and teeth to dissuade an enemy. He crouches and

restraint. When you consider restraining a cat, consider the maxim: *Less is more.* Although most cats object more strongly to being forcibly held down than the actual procedure you wish to accomplish, there are simply going to be times when a firm hold is required to get the job done and to prevent injury to the cat or the handler.

It is best to do most procedures on something that he's normally not allowed on, such as the kitchen table or bathroom vanity, as this puts him off guard. You'll have more control over the situation if you're working at waist level. Don't examine or treat your cat while he's lying on his favorite chair; he'll be much less cooperative than if you

Cross-legged restraint.

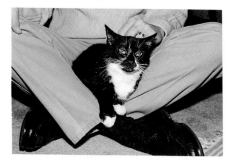

draws his limbs close to his body in preparation for springing. The fur stands erect to give the appearance that his body is larger than it really is. He lays his ears back flat and hisses convincingly with his mouth wide open.

If this posturing doesn't stop the confrontation, he strikes out with a front paw, or leaps forward to bite, and then retreats. Declawed cats tend to bite sooner when cornered. Up to this point, all the defensive behavior has been a warning. In true feline combat, a cat will wrap his front legs around his opponent and bite while raking with his back claws. Intervene and restrain your cat before any serious warnings are given.

Restraint Procedures

Scruffing

Your veterinarian or his assistant holds a less cooperative cat by the loose skin or *scruff* on the back of his neck. This is how a mother cat restrains and holds her kittens and in some cats this memory is very strong. Begin by giving your cat a friendly scratch on his forehead. Slide your dominant hand down the back of his neck and grasp as much of the loose skin there as you can between your fingers and palm. Cats tolerate this well, even if they've been restrained repeatedly this way; some cats become completely limp. Scruffing is not painful.

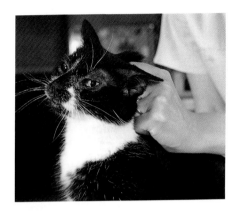

Your cat comes with a handle; it's called a "scruff."

If he does continue to struggle, give him a very slight shake, a quiver really, to remind him of the displeasure his mother showed to him and his unruly siblings.

Stretching

Once in a while a cat becomes very obstinate and scrappy when you hold onto his scruff. After all, it's so undignified and quite an affront to his self-esteem! Watch out for his back feet reaching forward to scratch. Use your other hand to grasp his back feet, just above the ankle or hock. Place one

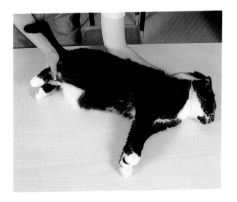

Stretching your cat prevents him from scratching you with his back feet, but you still need to watch out for his front claws.

STEP 1:
Lay your cat on the edge of the towel. Extend his legs back.

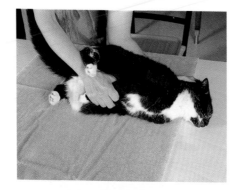

STEP 2:
Wrap the towel snugly around his neck and body to keep his legs in the drawn back position.

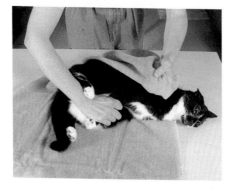

STEP 3:
Bring the other end of the towel up snugly as well.

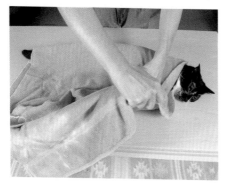

of restraint permits you to evaluate a good portion of the face and body. Have an assistant treat wounds or administer topical medications or insert a thermometer.

Towels and Cat Bags

Very fat cats don't have much of a scruff because the loose skin over the neck is taken up by stored fat. Frightened cats or muscular tomcats tighten their shoulders and shorten their neck, which also eliminates the scruff. And then there are some cats that will absolutely not tolerate scruffing under any circumstances. I have seen cats like this escape the grasp of an experienced veterinary technician and climb a bare wall.

To restrain any of these cats, roll them up in a thick bath towel. Wrap the cat with his front legs straight down and close to his body so that he can't reach forward to scratch. Pillowcases are handy for this type of restraint, but they're rarely strong enough to stand up to shredding by back claws. A canvas sack called a "cat bag" fits around the cat's body and leaves the head exposed. It's equipped with strategically placed zipper openings for access to limbs.

Hoods

A hood fits over the face and eyes and leaves an opening for the nose. A hood provides a comfortable darkness and sense of invisibility to the cat and functions as a muzzle if properly fit. A hood should be put on for as short a time as possible.

finger between each paw for a better grip. Then lay him on his side and stretch him out to a comfortable, relaxed length. Support his back with your forearm. This form

Trimming Claws

Trimming your cat's claws is another step in preventing injury to the handler. Ask your veterinarian or animal health technician to show you how during a routine examination and vaccination appointment. There are several different types of commercial nail clippers for animals. They can be purchased for less than ten dollars at a pet supply store or at your veterinarian's office. Choose the one you like best. Some nail trimmers have a replaceable blade. Animals don't mind having their nails trimmed as much if the blade is sharp. Alternatively, a pair of folding nail trimmers for people works very well for kittens and most adults, less so for a big ornery tomcat or very old cat with coarse nails.

You'll probably have to have an assistant scruff or stretch your cat in order to get him to cooperate for a nail trim. Gently hold the last joint of one toe between your thumb and forefinger. Squeeze the joint and see the claw flex outward. Clip off the sharp tip, avoiding the pink center, called the "quick," which bleeds if the nail is cut too short. Repeat for each claw. If the blade is dull, the end of the nail will appear ragged rather than smooth. If you do cut a claw too short, the bleeding will stop if you apply continuous pressure to the end of the nail for about a minute. Styptic powder (Kwik-Stop) or silver-nitrate applica-

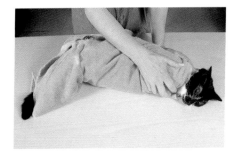

A kitty papoose.

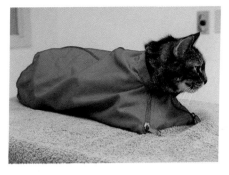

Cat bag restraint.

tor sticks act as a chemical cauterization but do cause a burning sensation. They are available at pet stores. A dab of flour or an ice cube held on the end of the nail works just as well.

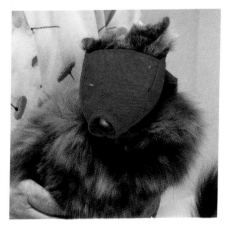

A hood or mask can have a quieting effect and help to prevent the handler from being bitten.

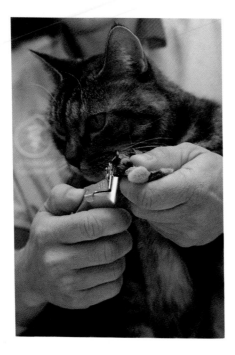

Trim off the sharp points but avoid the pink "quick" that contains blood vessels and nerves.

Check for an extra claw within the web of what would be the equivalent of our thumb. Because these claws are rudimentary, a cat can't push them out as he can with a fully developed one. When the new nail grows in, the cat can't remove the old one by digging it into wood, cloth, or your expensive leather couch. The old nail is instead pushed forward and becomes embedded in the soft web or pad, which is painful and can

become infected. This often happens in very old cats who don't take care of themselves. If you trim the nails of an old cat's claws you'll notice that you have to peel away the remnants of the old nail to see a tiny new one beneath it. If you discover an embedded nail, pain, a foul odor or discharge from your cat's toes, have your cat examined and the nails trimmed by your veterinarian. There are a variety of diseases with clinical signs such as these.

Whatever method or combination of methods you use to restrain your cat, use the minimum amount of necessary force to get the job done. If you're working with an assistant, decide how you're going to do it before you start. You'll only have one chance with some cats and any indecision on your part will give him the advantage and opportunity for escape. Make the restraint procedure as minimally displeasing as possible to insure his continued cooperation in the care-giving process. Under no circumstances should you hit your cat. *Physical punishment never results in cooperation.* If you're having difficulty getting your cat to cooperate, call your veterinarian. He will demonstrate restraint procedures safely and suggest alternatives.

Chapter 5
Keeping Records

Wellness Records

My cat Willie was born in an animal shelter 13 years ago and she's the only cat I've ever had that I actually went out and intentionally adopted. (The other two went out and adopted me.) Willie has moved with me to at least two dozen places and has crisscrossed this continent several times. She can claim something few cats can claim and that is to have been to the summit of Rocky Mountain National Park.

There's a lot to be said for keeping a record for healthy cats like Willie. If you move often, the information will help your new veterinarian be informed about your cat's past medical problems. A knowledge of past problems can hold the key to diagnosis of a current illness.

Travel across some state and all national boundaries requires that you have a health certificate that declares your cat to be free of infectious diseases and lawfully inoculated against rabies. All airlines require this paperwork at the

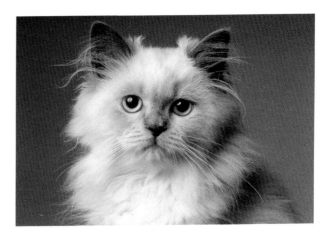

Have you seen this cat?

time of boarding. Health certificates are issued by your veterinarian. To obtain one, make an appointment for a physical examination. Bring your rabies certificate with you if the veterinarian issuing the health certificate is not the same one who administered the vaccine.

Table 2 lists some of the information that you should have available to you in your personal records for your cat. Aside from the medical record, have several good photographs of your cat to be used for identification if she is

**Table 2
Things to Include in Your
Cat's Wellness Record**

- Photographs
- Vaccination history
- Rabies certificates
- Health certificates
- Copies of medical records from previous veterinary hospitals or receipts for services
- Breeder's name and address
- Pedigree
- FeLV and FIV test results
- Results of stool analysis for parasites
- Your cat's normal body weight

ever lost. A photograph can be attached to a lost/found notice, photocopied, and posted in public places. Some owners make photograph postcards of lost pets and send them to veterinarians and animal shelters.

Questions Your Veterinarian May Ask

During an office call, your veterinarian is going to ask you some questions about your cat's behavior, the things she finds during the examination, and/or the problem at hand.

Table 3 lists some of the general questions she might ask. If you need

**Table 3
Questions Your Veterinarian
May Ask**

- Has your cat done any coughing or sneezing?
- Has he or she had any vomiting or diarrhea?
- Have you noticed any weight loss?
- How is your cat's appetite?
- How is your cat's attitude?
- What do you usually feed your cat? Have you changed foods and if so, when did you do this?
- Does your cat go outdoors?
- Are there any other animals at home? Are any of them ill?
- Can you think of anything your cat may have gotten into?
- When did you first notice a problem?
- Has the problem gotten worse, better, or stayed the same?
- How long has your cat had this problem?
- Has your cat ever had this problem before?
- Have you given your cat any medication for this problem and if so, what was it?
- If you think your cat has a fever, what is his or her temperature?

to drop your cat off at the hospital rather than schedule an appointment, write down as much information as accurately and as briefly as possible and include a phone number where you can be reached.

Using a Calendar

If you're giving your cat treatments at home or monitoring her progress, keep some brief notes about this too. Make a few mental or written notes to make sure that she's getting her medicine on time so you can accurately update your veterinarian. If your veterinarian asks you to check your cat's temperature during the day, do so and *write it down*. A calendar can help.

If your veterinarian sends home medication to be given two or three times a day, write the name of the medicine or the name of the cat and draw one line or box next to that name for every dose that is to be given during the day. Do this for every day that you're supposed to give the medicine. Under the box or line include the time each dose is to be administered if more than one person will be responsible for your cat.

Whenever your cat is given a pill, the person who does this can put a checkmark on the appropriate line or box. In this manner, everyone knows that she received her medicine. It will also remind you to finish out every prescription and will serve as a record so you can remember "the last time Fluff had this problem."

Some medications are prescribed on an every other day or every two day basis. When more than one drug is being given—for example, for cancer chemotherapy—calendars will help to keep track of cycles, as these types of drugs are given in patterns. Your veterinarian can help prepare and maintain the more complicated calendars in these cases.

MARCH 1–7						
Sunday 1	Monday 2	Tuesday 3	Wednesday 4	Thursday 5	Friday 6	Saturday 7
Little League 4 PM	PTA 7 PM	Fluff's pill ☐ 6 AM ☐ 6 PM	Fluff's pill ☐ 6 AM ☐ 6 PM	Office lunch	Fluff's pill ☐ 6 AM ☐ 6 PM	Tami's Shower NOON
Fluff's pill ☒ 6 AM ☒ 6 PM	Fluff's pill ☐ 6 AM ☐ 6 PM			Fluff's pill ☐ 6 AM ☐ 6 PM		Fluff's pill ☐ 6 AM ☐ 6 PM
103.5°F (39.7°C)	102.0°F (38.9°C)	101.5°F (38.6°C)	101.5°F (38.6°C)			

Other important information to record includes body temperature, appetite, water intake, bowel movements or diarrhea, urination, and overall attitude. Now when your veterinarian calls you can report with confidence: "Fluff's temperature was 101.5°F (38.6°C) all day yesterday, she had all her medicine, ate and drank normally, and doesn't have diarrhea anymore!"

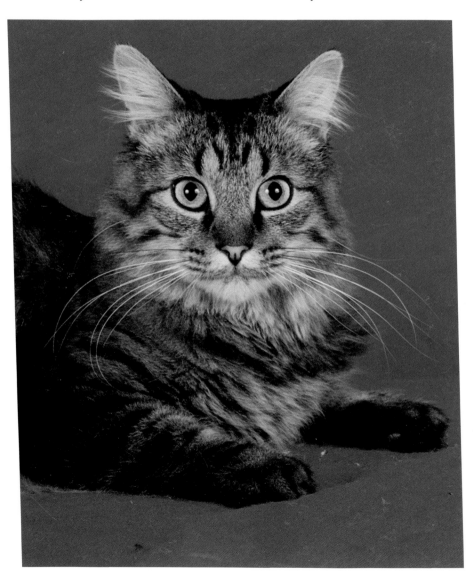

Chapter 6
The Sick Room

Adjusting to the Return Home

You can probably predict with some certainty how your cat will behave when he returns home after a day or two at the animal hospital. A lot of cats will disappear into the woodwork—you know they're in the house somewhere, peering at you from some invisible sanctuary. Other cats will curl up on their favorite chair or bed and catch up on the sleep they missed. Some sleep while others purr gratefully under an attentive eye. Mine enter, then eat.

The degree to which you watch over your convalescing cat depends upon the extent of his illness and the specific instructions given to you by your veterinarian. If you have a multiple cat household, reintroduce the patient to the stay-at-homes with some discretion. Even the best of feline pals hiss and torment the one who returns smelling like the animal hospital. Remind any children that the cat isn't feeling very well and to let him decide just how much human attention he's feeling up to.

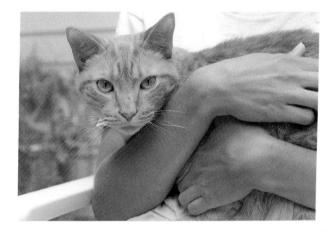

Confinement

Confinement within the home for all or part of the day is usually sufficient for most convalescing cats. If there is a question as to whether kitty will cooperate and use the litterbox, confine him to one room with a door that closes, like a bedroom or bathroom. Baby gates are a limited deterrent to roaming the house. I know this from personal experience. The cat will sit behind the gate, humoring me, and then effortlessly sail over the top when my back is turned just to prove a point.

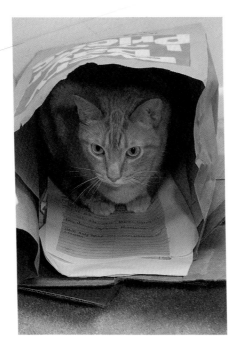

pools can be used, depending on the circumstances and the determination of the cat. Be creative.

Disgraceful as it may seem, cats often sleep inside their litterbox while confined to a cage. To discourage this, we give them a second litter tray, or a small box or dishpan as a bed. Line the box with an unwashed article of clothing that belongs to your cat's favorite person. If he can't use his back legs to stand or walk, turn the box so he can crawl inside. Check the bed frequently for urine and feces in case he doesn't move out of the bed to use the litterbox.

Litterboxes and Fillers

Cats with fractures, spinal injuries and severely ill cats must be strictly confined. Most cats who are this ill tolerate the confinement very well. Sometimes it is just a matter of finding a cage or a location for the cage that is acceptable to the cat. For instance, your cat may wail about being placed in a cardboard box in a back bedroom but be perfectly content in a more central location in the house.

Ask your veterinarian if you may borrow a portable cage or a large airline carrier. Many hospitals loan these out for free or with a deposit. If you have a friend with a large dog, ask if they have a large crate. Playpens, bathtubs, appliance boxes, laundry baskets, dishpans, or small wading

Use a regular litterbox for elimination if there is room in your cage. In the hospital we use disposable styrofoam or paper picnic plates equipped with about two tablespoons of cat litter; these are changed after each use. This conserves space and is more hygienic and pleasant for the cat, who would otherwise be confined inside a small compartment with a smelly litterbox.

The choice of cat box filler depends upon whether or not your cat has stitches and whether or not he insists on sleeping inside the litterbox despite your encouraging him to do otherwise. Sand and clay substances are unsuitable if your cat has an incision and sleeps in the box. The small particles stick to the wound and promote infection. Shredded newspaper or processed cellulose-type (yesterday's newspaper) cat box fillers are much less likely to enter the wound and promote infection.

Changing the type of filler can be a tricky thing with cats, as it can trigger an aversion to the box and inappropriate urination and defecation around the house. You and your veterinarian must weigh the risks of infection versus the risks of creating a litterbox problem.

Your veterinarian will have discharge instructions regarding diet, medication, at-home treatments, confinement, and need for rechecks. Go over these instructions with the individual who is responsible for discharging your cat from the hospital and ask them to clarify any point on which you are unsure.

When your cat comes home, allow him to find the place where he is most comfortable until the adjustment is made and his patterns of eating and sleeping are back to normal. Keep an eye on his appetite, water consumption, bowel movements and urination, and give him his medication if it has been prescribed. Keep your veterinarian informed of his recovery.

Heat Sources

There are a number of ways to provide an external heat source if your cat's body temperature is low.

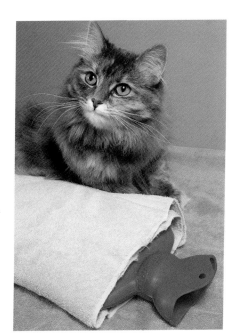

Containers filled with hot water are the safest method for raising the temperature near or around your cat. If you don't have a hot water bottle, fill any sealable container or some party balloons. Water-filled balloons can be microwaved for a few seconds to reheat.

Hot Water Bottles

The safest method is to fill a sealable container with hot water, wrap it in a soft towel, and place it in his bed. Use a hot water bottle if you have one, if not plastic soda bottles or water balloons do fine. Simply refill them when the water cools off or microwave them back to the proper temperature.

Heating Pads

There are two kinds of heating pads, those that heat up from an electrical current and those that heat with circulating hot water. Circulating hot water pads are safer because they maintain a more steady temperature, but they are very expensive, costing up to several hundred dollars apiece.

Don't allow your cat to lie on a heating pad if he can't or won't move off of it. Use hot water bottles instead, or attach the pad to the side of his bed or box with clothespins so that he doesn't have direct contact with it. Heating pads can cause serious burns that may not be apparent for several days.

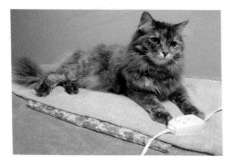

Electrical heating pads tend to fluctuate in temperature. Regardless of the setting, the temperature rises to surprisingly high levels on most commercial models while in use.

Heating pads are dangerous. Very sick cats tend to stay in one position and will not necessarily move off a heating pad if it gets too hot. If the cat is severely injured, it may not be able to move off even if

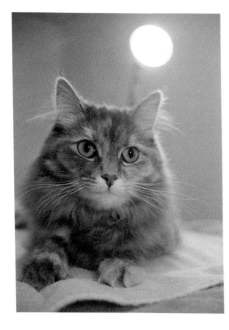

Use a heat lamp to warm the surrounding air. Don't point it directly on your cat.

it wanted too. Always put several layers of towel between your cat and the pad. Make sure he has room enough to move off the heating pad if he wishes, and is capable of doing so. *Never put the setting higher than low.*

Lamps

Lamps can also be used to provide heat. These are very effective, but their use carries the same risk of burns as do heating pads. Keep heat lamps positioned high above your cat's bed, and be sure he is able to move away from the lamp if he wants to.

Incubators

Another way to warm up your cat is to use an incubator. An aquarium works very well for this purpose. Cover the bottom with a soft towel. Place a heating pad inside the aquarium against one of the sides and use clothespins or the clips used for closing cereal boxes or snack bags to hold the heating pad in place. Alternatively, set the aquarium on top of the heating pad, with a towel between the two. Partially cover the top of the aquarium with another towel to hold in the heat.

Set the heating pad on low. I use a regular indoor/outdoor thermometer inside the incubator to monitor the temperature. Incubators like this are wonderful for orphaned kittens. For these little ones, I like to put some warm water balloons under the towel for them to nestle against.

Chapter 7
Keeping Watch

When we think of disease in animals and humans, especially the young and vigorous, we expect to recognize it right away by the outward signs: lethargy or inactivity, lack of appetite, vomiting or diarrhea. However, illnesses don't always present themselves in such obvious ways. Slowly progressive infections and organ dysfunctions can be difficult to detect because of the body's physiological ability to adapt.

For example, it is possible for a cat to become progressively more and more anemic due to feline leukemia virus infection and to act completely like herself until the number of red blood cells in the circulation is about one-fifth of normal. This is because her body tissues can adapt over a long period of time to the lower amount of oxygen delivered by the blood. A cat that loses four-fifths of her red blood cells because of hemorrhage after being hit by a car is not likely to survive, because the brain, heart, and kidneys are suddenly without oxygen.

A cat's stoic disposition and high tolerance to pain can also mask an illness. That's why your powers of observation are very important to the diagnosis and recovery of your cat. Your ability to account accurately for your cat's changes in appetite, bowel habits, and activity will assist your veterinarian in making a diagnosis, deciding on a course of therapy, and assessing whether your cat is responding to treatment.

Body temperature, heart rate and respiratory rate are collectively termed "vital functions," and are assessments of an animal's state of health. A single measurement of any one of these has limited value, but several measurements over hours or days can tell us a lot. Alternating high and low values, called cycles, may correspond among other things to the onset of pain, irregular heart rhythms, or release of bacteria or other substances into the blood. Cycles may determine when blood samples for certain laboratory tests should be drawn or when medications should be administered. So if your veterinarian asks you to monitor any of these vital signs, follow the recommended schedule as best you can, and write down your findings.

Body Temperature

Feeling the ears or fur for warmth is not an accurate method of determining your cat's body temperature, although a lot of people bring me their cat and tell me she has a fever because "she feels hot." Granted, a very high fever will make a cat's ears and fur feel warm, but so will the patch of sunlight or the waterbed on which your cat has been sleeping! To accurately measure body temperature, use a rectal thermometer, either a regular glass-mercury type or a digital model from a drug store.

With a standard rectal thermometer—shake down the mercury to a level below 96°F (35.6°C).

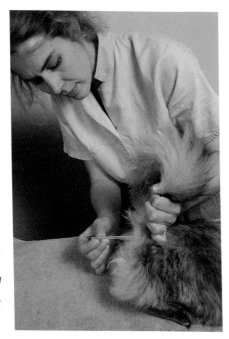

Learning to check your cat's body temperature is a very important skill that you can learn. Use some form of restraint, either scruffing or stretching by an assistant to make it easier.

Lubricate the bulb with a small amount of petrolatum or K-Y jelly. Lift your cat's tail and insert the tip of the thermometer into the anus. Push the thermometer forward at an angle approximately parallel to the spine until it is inserted about halfway. If you meet resistance, apply gentle, firm pressure, rotating the tip or modifying the angle until the anal sphincter relaxes and the insertion is complete. Leave the thermometer in place for 1½ to 2 minutes. Protect the thermometer from breaking by holding it in place or cupping your hand around it. Should it break, don't try to remove the fragment. Your cat will probably expel it herself within a short time. Call your veterinarian and let her know the situation, as kitty may need some professional assistance.

The newer digital thermometers have the advantage of being unbreakable. They come with disposable, prelubricated plastic sheaths to protect the probe and make cleaning easier. Follow the instructions for use that comes in the package, as thermometers may differ slightly between manufacturers. The process of insertion is the same as for a glass thermometer.

Some cats show very little resistance to having their temperature checked, at least for the first time! Kittens, cantankerous tomcats, and those with experience with the procedure frequently object to such an indignity. You might have to have an assistant scruff or stretch your cat to prevent injury and gain her cooperation.

The normal body temperature of a cat is 100.5° to 102.5°F (38.0°–39.2°C). It may register higher if your cat is agitated when you check it. I have seen perfectly normal kittens register a temperature of 104°F (40°C) during a visit to the hospital for examination. Kittens less than three or four weeks of age cannot regulate their body temperatures well, and require close physical contact with their mother to stay warm. A body temperature of 96°F (35.6°C) is essential for normal digestion of milk.

Body temperatures consistently above normal are classified as fever and this tells us that there is *inflammation* somewhere in the body. Notice that I did not say *infection*, although an infection will certainly result in inflammation. Any form of tissue damage will result in inflammation: trauma, surgery, poison, organ failure or dysfunction, cancer, or again, infection.

A fever can be a very necessary part of the healing process. Not all fevers are bad. The inflammation associated with surgery is essential to the healing process and often causes a low-grade fever. Fever also prevents the growth of some viruses and bacteria in the body and is therefore a natural defense against disease. That's why antipyretics and antibiotics are not appropriate in all instances of fever. Antibiotics are used to kill bacterial infections. If a

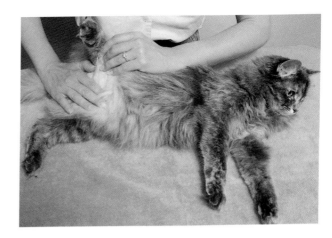

fever results from a viral infection, trauma, or surgery, antibiotics may or may not be an appropriate part of your cat's therapy.

This is a ticklish spot!

Very low body temperatures are usually a grave sign. The inability to maintain a normal body temperature is abnormal in all cats except very young kittens, and requires the immediate attention of your veterinarian.

Pulse and Heart Rate

A pulse is created by a wave of blood as it flows inside a blood vessel. The rhythmic pulse occurs every time the heart beats and pushes the blood forward through the arteries. It is easiest to feel at the arteries that are just under the skin, usually at the femoral artery located on the inside of the thigh. Naturally, detecting the pulse here

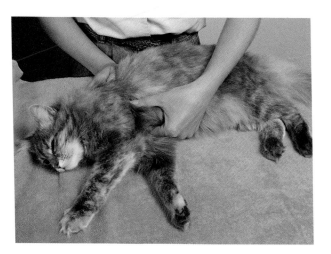

Feeling for a heart beat.

or anywhere can be very difficult in fat cats! If you place your fingertips on the inside of your cat's upper leg close to the body and move them back and forth, you will feel a thin, cordlike structure. Apply a very light touch and you will feel a slight pulsation. This takes practice!

It's much easier to feel the heart beating through the chest wall than to feel the pulse. Hold the chest between your thumb and fingers at the point where the elbow would touch it if it were flexed. To measure the pulse or heart rate, count the number of pulsations of the femoral artery or the heartbeats you feel in 15 seconds and multiply that number by 4. This is roughly the number of beats per minute. The normal value in a cat ranges from 120 to 200 depending on how excited he is.

Compare the numbers that you calculate for pulse and heart rate. They should be the same. In reali-

ty, the pulse rate is very difficult to measure even in a normal cat because it is usually so fast and so faint that only veterinarians and veterinary technicians have enough experience to make an accurate count.

The character of the pulse, its strength along with its approximate rate, can be a more important assessment of the circulatory system. Pulse character will be influenced both by how strongly the heart beats and by blood volume. For example, animals in shock due to blood loss (hemorrhage) will have a rapid and weak pulse because the heart is beating very fast in order to pump a reduced volume of blood through the circulatory system. The amount of blood moved by each heart beat is smaller than normal because the heart chambers don't have very much time to fill between beats. Marked differences in the pulse rate and heart rate are very noticeable, and herald circulatory failure.

In most instances, all your doctor will need to know is whether you can detect any pulse at all, either as a sign of life or as a sign of circulatory failure, usually at the rear limbs in cats.

Respiration

A breath is defined as one inspiration and one expiration. The number of breaths per minute is

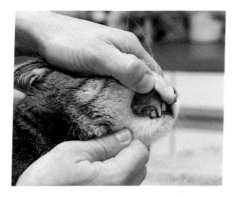

called the respiratory rate. This is measured by counting the number of times your cat's chest moves in and out in 15 seconds and multiplying that number by 4. In a quiet, sleeping cat this value may be around 30 breaths per minute. In an agitated cat or a cat in pain, it may be around 100 breaths per minute, so you see, like the pulse and heart rate, there is a wide range of "normal."

Here again, a more useful assessment of respiration is its character. Inhalation should be an easy movement of the chest outward and exhalation a gentle movement inward, lasting approximately three times longer. Cats experiencing respiratory distress will often have a prolonged inspiration, where the time it takes to inhale is as long or longer than the time it takes to exhale. Cats with breathing difficulties sometimes exhale with greater effort and use their abdominal muscles to "lift or push" air out of their lungs. Cats with respiratory diseases will con-

sistently have respiratory rates near 100 breaths per minute.

Do cats pant? Yes they do, usually when frightened or in pain, for instance in the car or in the examination room. The act of panting is not the same as breathing. During panting, air is moved back and forth in the larger airways. Little air is exchanged deep inside the lungs where oxygen is taken in by the blood and carbon dioxide is given up. Panting is also a means of exchanging heat since cats cannot sweat except from the bottoms of their paws.

Color

As a veterinarian, I probably see more puzzled looks on people's faces when I tell them that their cat is looking a little pale than when I

This cat's gums are pink and healthy.

This cat is icteric or jaundiced due to liver disease. Note the bright yellow pigmentation of the gums.

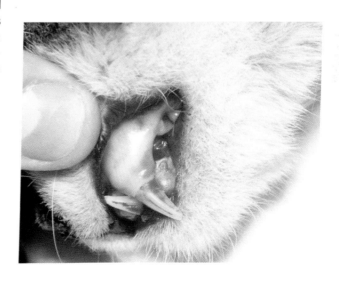

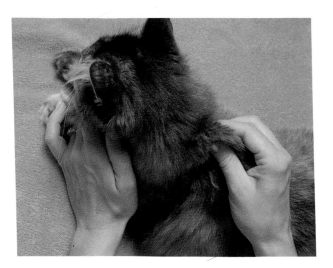

tell them anything else. Here sits a jet black cat or ruddy-red tabby and the doctor says, "She's looking a little pale!" ("I do trust Dr. Himsel, but she doesn't look like she's faded any to me...")

Now there are conditions that will change the color of the haircoat, but when we talk about color, veterinarians are really talking about the color of the mucous membranes—that is, the gums, the delicate tissues surrounding the eyes, lips, vulva, and prepuce. These tissues are not normally pigmented black (except in some cats, especially red tabby varieties as they age), and in the healthy cat, they look pink. Loss of that nice pink color is called pallor; it means your cat is pale and suggests the condition of anemia or a low red-blood-cell count. Anemia is not a disease, but rather a clinical sign of a disease process and warrants further investigation.

The sclera, or white portion of the eye, and the inside of the ear are also areas that your veterinarian will examine for color change. These tissues can turn yellow when there is a high level of a substance called bilirubin in the blood. Bilirubin is formed from the hemoglobin when red blood cells break down. When these tissues absorb the bilirubin and turn yellow, the cat is said to be *jaundiced* or *icteric*. This can be a sign of liver disease or a massive destruction of red blood cells.

It takes some practice to be able to recognize pale mucous membranes or icterus from the normal cat. If your cat has this problem, your veterinarian can compare your cat to a normal one so you can appreciate the difference.

Hydration

Water is the single most important nutrient required in the diet. Living creatures have developed a variety of adaptations in order to conserve water, and some are better at it than others. Cats, originating in the desert, conserve water far better than we do as humans.

Body water is normally lost in sweat, urine, feces, and breath. Prolonged, intense vomiting or diarrhea, lack of appetite, failure to drink, excessive urination, fever, and hemorrhage are all factors that put an animal's powers to conserve water to the test. Adult cats can tolerate water loss much better than kittens. Correcting dehydration and maintaining normal water balance is probably the single most important part of treatment for the ailing cat. Your veterinarian will administer intravenous or subcutaneous fluids based on the degree of dehydration and the underlying illness.

To evaluate for dehydration, feel your cat's gums. They should be moist and slippery. Lift the skin over the nape of her neck or her scruff; it should fall back down right away. In the dehydrated cat, the gums will be tacky and the skin over the neck will stand up like a tent or fall very slowly back to normal. Weight loss of a pound or two over a day or so also signals dehydration.

Collecting Fecal Samples

For most routine examination of the stools for parasites, a sample of feces about the size of a walnut is all your veterinarian will need. If your veterinarian will be examining the specimen for microscopic larvae, she will need about three or four times that amount. The sample should be as fresh as possible, no more than 24 hours old at the time of examination. If you can't bring it in to the hospital right away, place the sample in the refrigerator. If the veterinarian is looking for *Giardia*, a protozoal parasite, the sample should be fresh but not refrigerated.

The sample can be collected in a small jar or a plastic bag. Some veterinarians will give you a small container in which the stool will be analyzed, so that no one has to handle the feces after it is collected. A small amount of kitty litter or dirt in the sample is not a problem. If your cat's feces are being examined because of diarrhea, blood, or mucus, try to provide a representative sample of the abnormal stool.

Collecting Urine Samples

Your veterinarian may request a urine sample from your cat for analysis of such substances as glucose and ketones if she is diabetic, or for blood, crystals, proteins, and the cellular components. If the sample is not to be cultured for bacteria, a sample "caught" at home is sometimes requested. The easiest

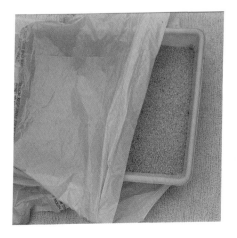

To collect a urine sample, fill the litterbox with litter and place inside a large kitchen garbage bag.

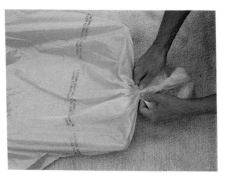

Pat out the air and close with a twistie tie. if your litterbox has a cover, replace it. Samples collected in this manner can't be used for urine culture because they will be contaminated by bacteria from the environment and thus yield false results. They can, however, be used for routine urinalysis.

way to catch a urine sample is to place a nonabsorbent material over the litter. Some cats will comply nicely if you just put a piece of foil or plastic over the box; however, your cat may miss if her target is too small or you may spill the sample during retrieval.

One sure-fire method of catching urine is to place litter in the box as you normally would and then to place the whole box, contents and all, inside a tall kitchen garbage bag. Flatten out the air, close the bag with a twistie tie and return the box to its original location. Your cat can now feel the texture of the litter under her feet. Most cats will readily use the box. Use a syringe to aspirate the urine from the plastic, and then squirt it into a scrupulously clean jar or container provided by your veterinarian. If you are checking for urine sugar and ketones yourself at home, proceed as instructed. If you are transporting the sample to the hospital, refrigerate it if it will be delayed. Be aware that refrigeration can cause changes in the urine and misleading results in some tests. If your cat has a lot of "flea dirt" in her fur that drops off into the sample, the analysis for blood can also be inaccurate. Flea dirt is flea excrement, and consists of blood sucked from your cat. An alternative method of collection by your veterinarian will be necessary to eliminate these factors that can cause misinterpretation of the tests.

Chapter 8
Feeding and Nutrition

General Nutrition

L et's begin by looking at the six major nutrients, and their functions within the body: *carbohydrates, proteins, fats, minerals, vitamins*, and the most important one, *water*.

Three of the six major nutrients can be used by the body to produce the chemical energy needed to power life processes and heat. The heat released when these nutrients are "burned" by the body is measured in calories. Carbohydrates and proteins release approximately 4 kcals or calories per gram weight. Fats contain more than twice as many calories at 9 kcals per gram weight.

Carbohydrates

Carbohydrates come from plant sources: grains, seeds, vegetables, and grasses. Carbohydrates can be simple in their chemical structure, like sugar, or complex, like cellulose. Cellulose and other similar complex carbohydrates make up the physical structure of plants. Some of these complex carbohydrates cannot be digested by animals, and are then labeled *dietary fiber*. Although it is not digested, fiber plays an important role in normal intestinal function.

Proteins

Proteins are not one substance, but many substances made up of smaller subunits called amino acids that are linked together. Proteins make up all the tissues and fluids of animals; they serve a structural

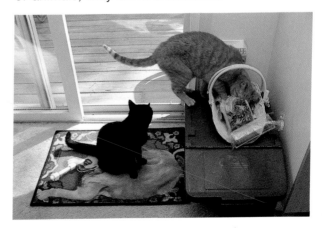

role. Proteins also function as hormones and chemical transmitters within nerves. The sequence and arrangement of the amino acids in a protein determines the function of that protein.

Proteins are not derived solely from animal tissue; they are also available from plants. Once consumed by an animal, digestion breaks protein down into its constituent amino acids, then they are absorbed into circulation and recombined into structural proteins needed by the animal. Animals can make amino acids on their own, but not all of them. Although there are 23 amino acids, cats require that 11 of them be provided by the diet. Twelve others can be synthesized in the body.

Taurine is one amino acid that is required in the cat's diet, but not in the dog's. This amino acid is critical for normal heart function and vision. *Arginine* is another amino acid required in much higher amounts by cats. Arginine is essential for converting the waste product ammonia into urea, so that it can be excreted by the kidneys. Insufficient arginine levels can cause depression and seizures.

No single protein contains all 23 amino acids. That means that a cat must eat several different sources of protein in order to obtain all eleven of the essential ones. The proteins from meat contain a greater variety of amino acids than do proteins from plants. The word "biologic value" is used to describe the completeness of a protein's complement of amino acids. Eggs are almost perfect and have a biologic value of 98, while corn rates a BV of 45 and beef a BV of 78. This concept of biologic value becomes important as we talk about how cat foods are developed.

Proteins also have *bioavailability* characteristics. Broken down, the word refers to *bio* or life, and *availability*, meaning accessible. Proteins with high bioavailability are easily digested and utilized by the body and little of this protein is eliminated in the feces. The opposite is also true. Intuitively we can see that although feathers, hooves, and animal hides are all made up of tissue and therefore proteins, they will not be as digestible and utilizable as protein derived from skeletal muscle. The protein from animal hides is more likely to be lost in the feces.

All 23 amino acids must be present and available in order for the body to synthesis proteins. That means that if a cat or other animal takes in a meal that is deficient in any one amino acid, protein synthesis stops. The available amino acids are then burned for energy. Excess energy is stored as fat, and ammonia is released as a waste product. The same holds true if protein is consumed in excess amounts from what is needed to manufacture the body's structural proteins. This becomes very important in diseases like obesity and kidney disease, as we shall see.

Protein, in fact, is a very questionable and controversial energy source, and in most healthy animals should be avoided in excess. The cat is unique among animals, however, because the cat is one species that actually requires some of its energy to come from protein. This is one reason why cats require more protein in their diet than dogs. The reason for this species difference is not known, and because of the cats' additional requirement for the animal-tissue-derived amino acid taurine, they are true obligate carnivores. This is an important point. Cats should not be fed dog food.

Fats

Fats serve several functions within the body. First, they are a highly efficient source of energy (9 kcals/gram). Fats are also necessary for the absorption of some vitamins: vitamins A, D, E, and K. They are also important in the formation of certain hormones. Fats are similar to proteins in that they are made up of subunits called fatty acids. Two of the essential fatty acids for the cat are required in their diet: *linoleic* and *arachidonic*.

Just as there are different qualities of proteins, some fats are better than others in providing essential fatty acids. Fats can be found in both vegetable matter and animal tissue. Liquid fats like safflower oil and corn oil consist of 50 to 70 percent linoleic acid. Arachidonic acid is found only in animal fats. A cat's requirement for arachidonic acid in the diet makes it a truly carnivorous animal. Poultry fat is an excellent source of arachidonic acid. This is an expensive ingredient in pet foods, so most manufacturers use an alternative called beef tallow, which is less expensive but a relatively poor source of essential fatty acids.

Diets high in fat, or those that contain poorly preserved fat that has gone rancid, put cats at risk for a disease called *pansteatitis*. Even properly formulated, high-quality diets that have been stored for long periods of time or at high temperatures should not be fed to cats. Toxins present in rancid fats can accumulate in the cat's own subcutaneous fat stores along the back or in that udderlike fat pad that sways to and fro when they walk. These toxins set up an inflammation that is self-perpetuating and very, very painful. Fortunately, this isn't very common. Most afflicted cats have been eating a fish diet.

Since the fish in cat foods comes from the by-products of the human canned-fish industry, the quality of the ingredients is highly questionable. In fact, fish is not even a natural part of a cat's diet! I have never once heard of a cat leaving a fish on the doorstep, as a gift to its owner. Indeed, the need for fish in the cat's diet has solely—no pun intended—come from the advertising and pet-food industries.

Vitamins

Vitamins can be divided into two groups: those that will dissolve in water and those that will dissolve in fat. Vitamins that dissolve in water are called *water soluble*, and these are the various B vitamins and vitamin C. These vitamins are not stored in the body to any extent and become rapidly depleted during periods of inappetence. Vitamins that dissolve in fat are called *fat soluble*. These include vitamins A, D, E, and K. They dissolve in dietary fat and, with the assistance of bile, are then absorbed as the fats are absorbed. These vitamins are then stored within the fatty tissues of the body.

Vitamins are used in the energy-producing reactions of the body. They are important in wound healing, tissue repair, maintaining healthy skin, haircoat and bones, and in blood clotting. Many animals, including dogs and people, can synthesis some vitamins—for example, vitamin A can be synthesized from betacarotene, the substance that gives carrots their orange color. The B vitamin called niacin can be synthesized from biotin. This is not true, however, for cats. Cats require both vitamin A and niacin in their diet. These vitamins are found in animal tissues and again, their requirement makes the cat a truly carnivorous animal. Because cats have different requirements for the levels of vitamins in their diet, they should not be fed dog food.

Vitamin deficiencies are rarely a problem in healthy cats eating a wholesome diet. Deficiencies can occur if a cat is fed a poorly formulated diet or food that is improperly stored or preserved. Vitamins are subject to rapid degradation in high temperatures during the cooking process. This is most often the case with generic or very inexpensive cat foods and with home cooked diets. Improperly processed fish cat foods may also contain a substance that destroys the B vitamin called thiamine. In the most severe form of thiamine deficiency, cats can develop depression and seizures.

Some disease conditions can result in a vitamin depletion. Because the water-soluble vitamins are not stored in the body, they will be depleted rapidly if a cat is allowed to go without food for even a few days, especially if the cat is losing a lot of water from kidney disease, vomiting, or diarrhea. Diseases that result in improper absorption of fats will of course effect the absorption of the fat-soluble vitamins too. Because fat soluble vitamins are in reserve, problems related to deficiencies in these vitamins usually occur after a longer period of time.

Vitamin excesses are potentially a problem when cats are being fed home-cooked diets. It is very difficult to balance these diets with the proper nutrient levels, because the batches are small and the vitamin sources are quite concentrated in comparison. Vitamin excesses are also a potential problem for cats who are given vitamin supplements in their diets or as treats. *Never give a vitamin supplement unless you are instructed to do so by your veterinarian.*

Minerals

Minerals serve as an important structural component in the body. Calcium, phosphorus, and magnesium make up the matrix of bones and teeth. Sodium and potassium are important in maintaining cell shape and in nerve conduction. Calcium is also needed for muscles to contract. Minerals such as iron and copper are needed for proper red-blood-cell function. Zinc is important for healthy skin.

Minerals are needed in trace amounts in the diet; they are provided by both plant and animal sources. However, most of the mineral in cat foods comes from bone meal and meat meal used in formulating the diets. Poor quality and cheap meat ingredients used in making cat food, have a lot of bone in them. This bone is expensive to remove from the meat scraps, so it is usually just left in. Most cat foods contain minerals in amounts that far exceed the requirements of the cat. This is especially true of fish-con-

taining diets. These excessive minerals have to be eliminated from the cat's body, usually in the urine.

Ash refers to the residue that is left when a diet is burned to completion. You can think of ash as being basically the same substance that is left on the bottom of your fireplace or in your wood stove after a nice Sunday afternoon with your cat in your lap and a good novel. Ash is a mineral residue. The name does not specify which minerals or how much of any one there may be in the mix.

Water

Although water is being talked about last, it is truthfully the most important of the six basic nutrients. Most animals cannot live more than a short time without it, or more than a few days without becoming dehydrated and sick. Water comprises from about 95 percent of the newborn animal to about 75 percent of the adult. (Now you know where the expression "You're all wet!" comes from.) Water is the body's primary solvent for chemical reactions and life processes, and maintains cell shape. Throughout the animal kingdom, animals have evolved elaborate adaptive mechanisms to conserve water. Of paramount importance in this role is the kidney. And cats, originally from the desert, are particularly efficient at conserving water and producing very concentrated urine.

In summary, cats are classified as true carnivores, that is they are true meat-eating animals because they must consume proteins and fats from animal-tissue sources. This is for several major reasons. First, the essential amino acid taurine and the essential fatty acid arachidonic acid are only present in animal tissue. Secondly, of the vitamins, cats cannot convert beta carotene from plants into vitamin A, nor can they convert biotin into the B vitamin called niacin. Both of these vitamins therefore must come from animal tissue. Cats, unlike dogs, require some of their energy to come from protein; they also have higher requirements for some specific amino acids and vitamins. For all of these reasons, cats should not be fed diets formulated for dogs.

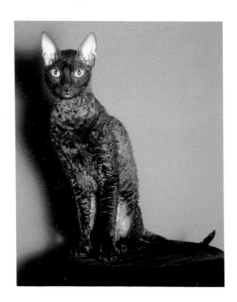

Choosing a Diet for a Healthy Cat

Pet ownership, like parenting, doesn't come with an owner's manual. Thus, when choosing a pet food, most people rely on advice and information that is readily available to them to make that decision: friends, family, past experience, books and pamphlets, a veterinarian's recommendation, and in most instances, what is said in advertising. One stroll down the pet food aisle in the grocery or pet store and you can quickly see that many of the claims made by pet-food companies are nonnutritional and nonscientific, and have little to do with providing a well-balanced, free-from-harmful-excesses diet for animals. Some examples of these claims include variety, kibble size, shape or color, convenience of packaging, flavor, and even how the product comes out of the can. Scientific claims for: highest level of nutrition and quality, meeting or exceeding government standards, or feeding trials, are largely unsubstantiated and misleading. Here are some features you should insist upon:

Fixed formulation. These foods are prepared using the same set of ingredients in every batch. Unless the label says "fixed formulation," you should assume that the manufacturer uses the ingredients that are the least expensive at the time. The FDA does not require that the label on a can or box be changed for six months. For this reason, what you see on the label may not actually be what is in the product.

Digestibility. Highly digestible diets mean that more nutrients are actually available to the cat. There is less waste to clean out of the litterbox, and your cat will eat less, which means it costs less to feed a highly digestible food. This is especially important for kittens. Kittens must consume much larger quantities of poorly digestible diets in order to obtain adequate calories and nutrients for growth and development, which may be impossible with their small stomach capacity.

Palatability. The most nutritious diet in the world is useless unless a cat will actually eat it. Fat, protein, salt, temperature, acidity or alkalinity, and texture are very important palatability factors for cats. These can be used to coax a cat to eat when he's not feeling well. Some of these factors can be very harmful—salt, for instance. On the other hand, just because a diet is palatable, that doesn't mean that it is nutritious or even good for your cat. As an example, diets made with beef tallow are very palatable to cats, but we know that beef tallow is a relatively poor quality source of essential fatty acids. Fish, also extremely palatable, contains potentially harmful excesses of minerals and possibly substances that destroy thiamine or cause pansteatitis.

Balanced for the particular stage in the cat's life. Nutrient requirements change depending upon the life stage of the cat. The energy and nutrient requirements for a growing kitten and pregnant queen are nearly double that of a nonpregnant adult cat. If a cat food is labeled "for all stages of growth and maintenance," you should be aware that that food is formulated to meet the greater needs of kittens and pregnant adults and could contain excessive amounts of nutrients that may be harmful to the nonpregnant adult cat and to cats with certain diseases that we will discuss later in this book.

Diets for Sick Cats

Sick cats require special considerations as to diet. For cats that continue to eat even in the face of an illness, their regular diet is probably fine, provided there is adequate caloric and nutrient intake, including water. You can monitor this by weighing your cat and noting any weight loss. An additional check on water intake is to test the skin turgor or hydration status (see page 50). The advantage of sticking with the same food is that there is less of a problem with vomiting or diarrhea that so often occurs with a change in diet.

Diet often plays a role in the treatment of disease in both human and veterinary medicine—you may have a family member who is on a sodium or cholesterol-restricted diet. We use research-based principles to control diseases in animals, too. Fortunately, rather than having to cook and balance homemade diets, there are scientifically formulated prepared canned, dry, and liquid foods available by prescription through your veterinarian. The importance of clinical nutrition in the recovery from disease cannot be overemphasized. In many situations, the dietary management used in treatment is as important or more important than the drugs. If you are advised by your veterinarian to use a specially formulated prescription-type diet, you should follow those instructions as closely as you would for giving medication.

Prescription-type diets are unlike any commercially available cat food. These diets should not contain unnecessary amounts of protein, fat, or salt to enhance the flavor as do most cat foods. These diets most likely do not have the same texture or "mouth-feel" as your cat's regular diet either, although many prescription-type diets are formulated in both a canned and dry form.

For these reasons, your cat may not willingly eat a prescription-type diet when it is first offered. This lack of cooperation is much the same problem that physicians have with patients instructed to change their eating habits significantly. Unfortunately, cats are even less open to reasoning than people.

Consult the following pages on assisted feeding for help with this task.

While home-cooked diets are very difficult to balance and are not advisable in the long run, sometimes it is necessary to prepare a special diet for your cat. This may be the case for a cat with a food intolerance that necessitates a very simple diet with few ingredients to be fed as a food trial. However, home-cooked diets are becoming increasingly unnecessary, as more and more prescription-type diets have been developed to meet a cat's special needs. If your veterinarian specifies a home-cooked diet, follow the recipe exactly. Do not substitute ingredients unless you check with the doctor first.

Assisted Feeding

My household doesn't need an alarm clock in the morning. We hear the dulcet tones of our white cat Neige calling for her breakfast. I tell you truthfully that she can say my name, for her "meow" sounds just like "kare-roll..." If she keeps it up long enough, I do respond. When any one of my cats doesn't appear for breakfast, I know something is amiss. It could be that Willie has just crawled into an open dresser drawer again, and sleeps among the sweaters with the drawer now closed! In my house failure to respond to the clatter of pouring cat food in the bowl or the can opener means someone is sick.

A lack of interest in food doesn't necessarily mean that your cat isn't feeling well. If your cat is of the outdoor variety, he may be eating at a benevolent neighbor's, or perhaps has recently dined on a meal of wild game. The finicky cat, one who turns up his nose at your offering, is a creature created by our own need to please. It is simple to prevent this behavior—just choose a well-balanced, high-quality food during kittenhood, and stick with it!

Variety in the diet is something that humans crave, but I have my doubts about cats. It is hard to believe that a mother cat, while teaching her kittens to hunt, would pass up a mouse just because they had that for dinner yesterday! And I seriously doubt that in the wild little mousies taste much different than little chipmunks or little birds.

You are the best person to judge whether your cat is just being finicky, or truly inappetant. A true lack of appetite, lasting longer than a day or two, probably signals illness and should not be ignored. It is better to have your veterinarian examine your cat early, than to wait a week or more and let the open cans of cat food pile up in your refrigerator. If you find yourself buying fresh swordfish to tempt your cat while serving tuna casserole to your family, call your veterinary hospital.

Cats that do not take in any food for 48 hours or more are at risk of developing a liver disease called *hepatic lipidosis* or *fatty liver syndrome*. The exact mechanism by which this disease develops is not completely understood. It probably relates to the cat's unique metabolism and liver physiology. Hepatic lipidosis results in the accumulation of fat in the liver which interferes with the function of the normal liver tissue. Obese cats that stop eating for any reason are particularly susceptible, but all cats can be effected.

Cats that are ill from other diseases—respiratory infections, wounds, injuries, cancers, etc.—should be made to eat as soon as possible. There are very few diseases where withholding food is important in treatment—vomiting and diarrhea may be two of these exceptions. Failure to provide adequate intake of nutrients, especially protein, will result in rapid weight loss and a very noticeable loss of muscle, because the cat will use its own body tissues for energy. Without protein, fats, carbohydrates, vitamins, minerals and water, the immune system cannot fight infection, wounds cannot heal, and nervous tissue, especially the brain, will not function properly. Antibiotics and other drugs cannot compensate for lack of food. Most medications work in concert with not independently of the immune and organ systems of the body for their intended effects.

Hand-feeding

With all that said, how do we go about getting a cat to eat? There are a variety of methods. Let's start with voluntary intake—this is the method most people use because it is obviously the easiest. You can make your cat's regular diet more palatable by warming it to room temperature or slightly above by microwaving or steaming. The addition of broth, either homemade or low-sodium canned type, to make a gravy will work too. The texture and how a food feels inside the mouth seems to be more important with cats than with other species. In other words, some cats prefer chunks of food, others prefer ground meat or purees. During illness, your cat's preferences may change from what it prefers when in good health.

Scrape a small amount of food onto your cat's hard palate and behind his top front teeth.

While normally I do not recommend top dressing a balanced cat food with cooked meats, baby foods, or cottage cheese, I make an exception if I need to get food into a sick cat. For top dressing, I prefer to use an already pureed, prescription-type diet made specifically for the purpose of feeding stressed or anorectic dogs and cats. You can obtain this diet from your veterinarian.

Putting the food in front of your cat and then stroking his head and neck can stimulate a cat to eat. Putting the first dollop into his mouth may be all your cat needs to continue on his own. You can also dab a little on his nose or paw and get him to lick it off. Some sick cats prefer to eat off a flat plate or out of your hand, instead of a bowl. If your cat seems to lose interest in canned food once it has been flattened to the walls of the bowl or edge of the dish, stir it up with a fork, back to your cat's preferred texture.

Syringe-feeding

If your cat will not voluntarily take in significant amounts of food, he can be force-fed by syringe. To do this, you can use a puree made with either your cat's regular cat food or a prescription-type diet, strained to remove the larger particles. There is a prescription-type diet already prepared in this form that is appropriate for most sick cats. Some veterinarians use liquid diets, either those

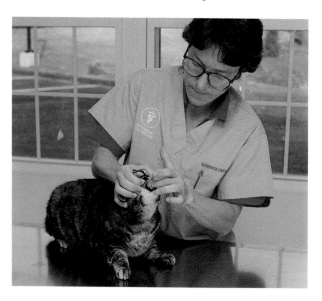

made for people and sold at pharmacies, or those made for veterinary patients. Personally I do not use these liquid diets often because they are messy to use and it is difficult to feed a cat a significant volume of the diet with a syringe. Still, your cat may be willing to lap a liquid diet from a bowl.

To syringe-feed your cat, draw up a manageable volume into an appropriate syringe. Your veterinarian will provide you with one of several types—either a smaller, regular syringe without a needle, used for injections, or a feeding syringe with a special tip that can be inserted into the mouth and towards the back of the tongue. Insert the syringe either directly into the front of the cat's mouth, or through the side in the space between the upper and lower jaw. Squirt a little bit into the mouth and allow your cat to swallow. Of course, you should only syringe-feed a cat that is fully conscious and capable of swallowing.

Tube-feeding

If adequate amounts of nutrition cannot be fed by hand or syringe, it is very appropriate to use a tube. Feeding tubes can be inserted and left in place for an indefinite period of time, or they can be inserted just for feedings, as is most often the case for newborn kittens. Tube-feeding can make all the difference

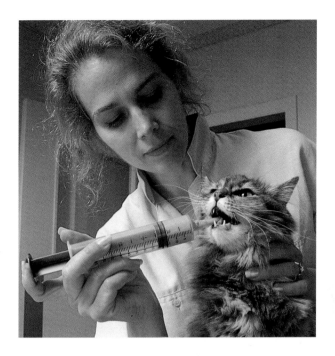

in the world to recovery, and you can have your cat at home, even with these tubes.

The simplest and least stressful type of feeding tube is one that is inserted in through the nose and down into the lower esophagus or stomach. Your veterinarian can do this using a few drops of a local anesthetic in the nostril in an already depressed cat, or with a light sedative. These tubes are then sutured into place over the bridge of the nose, avoiding the whiskers. A funnel-like barrier called an Elizabethan collar around the cat's neck will prevent him from taking the tube out. Sometimes a cat will sneeze this tube out, but replacing it is fairly easy. Because these

Syringe feeding works best using a semi-solid, pureed diet. Liquid diets dribble out the mouth and the cat actually consumes very little.

tubes have a very small diameter, a fairly liquid diet will be necessary. Larger feeding tubes can be placed through the cheek area and down the esophagus, or directly into the esophagus on the side of the neck. These feeding tubes require anesthesia and surgical placement, a procedure which will cost more. However, they can be used longer and are generally better tolerated by the cat. Also, the diet doesn't have to be as liquid in consistency, which means there is a greater flexibility in providing the most appropriate nutrition to the patient.

There is one more practical method of tube feeding that involves placement of a tube directly into the stomach. These tubes have been used in both humans and animals for months at a time. They require complete anesthesia and either a surgical procedure or the use of a special piece of equipment called an endoscope. Many veterinary hospitals now have endoscopes that allow examination of the stomach and other parts of the gastrointestinal or respiratory tracts, or else have access to hospitals or mobile veterinary services with endoscopes. These tubes do cost more than other types of feeding tubes, still, depending upon the circumstances of your cat, a gastrostomy (stomach) tube may be the best choice. Semi-liquid foods can be used with these.

For completeness sake, I will mention feeding tubes that by-pass the stomach and upper gastrointestinal tract and are inserted directly into the intestine itself. These tubes, called jejunostomy tubes, require anesthesia and surgical placement. Usually, these tubes are used only in the hospital under expert nursing care, and special liquid diets are necessary.

Regardless of the type of tube used, the procedure for tube-feeding is the same. In each case, have ready in the feeding syringe the amount of food you intend to feed. Squirt a small amount of tap water into the tube first, to make sure that the tube isn't plugged. Then slowly squirt in the diet you are using. Administer it slowly and watch for any signs of distress or potential vomiting. This usually isn't a problem unless you try and feed too much at one meal, or the cat has an intolerance to one of the ingredients in the diet. It helps to warm the diet to room temperature or slightly above. Once your cat has been fed, squirt enough tap water through the tube to clear it. Some veterinarians will have you cap the tube. If you have removed an Elizabethan collar or bandage in order to make the tube more accessible, be sure and replace it right away.

Feeding Newborn Kittens

These are some of my favorite patients! More of these patients have come home with me at the end of the day than any other. If the newborn kitten is in your care because of abandonment or the death of the mother, your job is probably going to be easier than if the kitten is failing to thrive under its own mother's care. For a more complete discussion on care of the newborn, see page 103.

Newborn kittens require a liquid diet that closely matches the nutrients of mother's milk. Such milk replacements are found in a powdered form that requires mixing with water, or in a can, already reconstituted. I prefer the powdered form because you can make it up fresh. These formulas require refrigeration and have a relatively short shelf-life when opened. You can purchase milk replacement from your veterinarian and from many pet stores.

When you purchase the formula, be sure to buy a pet nurser too. These look just like a doll's baby bottle and you'll need to cut a hole in the nipple. The biggest mistake most people make when they're bottle feeding kittens is to fail to make the hole big enough, so don't just pierce it with a pin, cut the end off!

As a starting point, follow the recommendations on the can for the volume of diet your kitten will need for one day. A rule of thumb is to feed the kitten as much as it will take every two to four hours. If that sounds vague, don't worry—your kitten will probably wake up and cry when it's time to eat! Most kittens

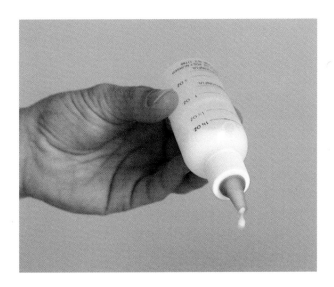

will not require any middle-of-the-night feedings.

To bottle-feed your kitten, warm approximately two ounces of fresh formula in a pan of warm water. Check the formula temperature on your wrist before feeding. It should be slightly warmer than room temperature. Avoid making the formula so warm that it could scald your kitten's digestive tract. Hold the kitten in the palm of your hand in an upright position rather than on its back. Most kittens will readily accept the nipple if you put it in their mouth. If it doesn't begin sucking right away, squeeze a few drops of formula into its mouth. If the kitten falls asleep, wiggle the bottle in his mouth a little to remind him of the task at hand.

Newborn kittens do not urinate or defecate on their own, but rely on their mother to stimulate these

The opening in the nipple is big enough if a drip forms when the bottle is inverted.

reflexes. The mother does this by licking under the kitten's tail. After every meal, you will need to stroke the kitten under the tail with a warm, wet cotton ball, to stimulate urination and defecation. Newborn kittens pass nearly colorless urine because it is very dilute, so watch closely for drops of urine to appear. The kitten's stool or feces will be very soft and light in color. If your kitten continues to cry inbetween meals, he may be constipated and require a gentle enema to get things moving along. You should bring the kitten to your veterinarian for this. Submerging the kitten's hindquarters in a warm-water bath will sometimes help too.

Kittens with a poor suckling reflex who fail to thrive will require tube-feeding. Your veterinarian will show you how to do this and give you the feeding tube and syringe. The first step is to measure and mark the tube so that you know how far to insert it. Mark the tube at the distance between the last rib and the tip of the nose. This puts the tube as far as the kitten's stomach. Your veterinarian will advise you as to the volume of formula to feed at each meal, and the frequency of the feedings. Have the formula warmed and drawn up into the syringe, all ready to go. Wet the end of the tube so that it will slide easier. Hold your kitten upright and push the tube into the back of his mouth. Most kittens will fuss a little at this point as the tube enters the

upper esophagus. Try to keep the kitten's head and neck held at a normal angle, rather than with the neck extended or flexed. This will make it easier to enter the esophagus, and avoiding accidentally entering the trachea or windpipe. Kittens will not necessarily cough if the tube enters the trachea.

The tube should easily enter the esophagus. If you encounter any resistance, withdraw the tube and try again. Your kitten may try and chew the tube as it is passed. Pass the tube into the stomach as far as the mark. Sometimes you can feel the end of the tube in the stomach. Attach the syringe to the end of the tube, and slowly push the plunger and give the formula. Do not feed too much or too fast, or your kitten may regurgitate and breathe in the formula. If the tube has accidentally entered the trachea, a small amount of formula in the lungs is not necessarily fatal, but is a grave problem. Fortunately, placing the tube in the trachea and lungs is harder than you think! You may be able to alternate tube feeding with bottle feeding. As your kitten becomes stronger, tube feeding will become unnecessary.

At about three weeks of age, when your kitten's eyes and ears open and he begins to explore his environment, begin to mix warm milk replacement with a canned kitten-growth-formula diet on a flat plate. When he begins to cry for food, put the plate in front of him and push his little face into it. At first he'll probably suck out the liquid. If he doesn't catch on, just bottle feed as usual. After a day or two he'll probably get the idea and begin to take mouthfuls of slurry. Over a couple of weeks, gradually reduce the amount of milk replacement until he's eating solid food. Don't rush this process. You can begin to offer a dry kitten-growth diet at about eight weeks of age.

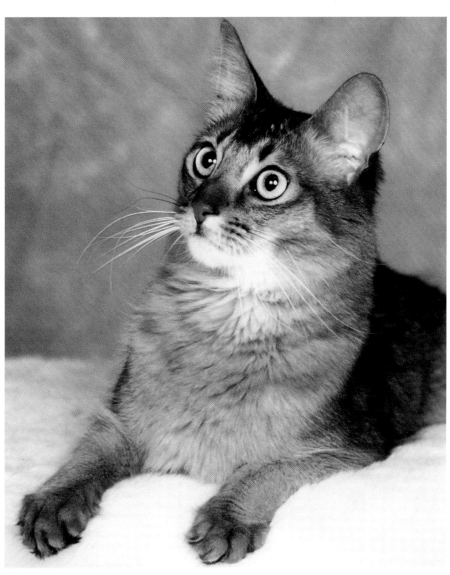

Chapter 9

Medications and Prescriptions

General Information

Most but not all of the medication that you will ever give your cat will be a veterinary preparation provided by your veterinarian, who maintains a pharmacy within the hospital. Sometimes you'll have to have a prescription filled at a drugstore, especially if your cat needs a medicine that your veterinarian doesn't keep in stock. In this case, the doctor can call the pharmacist and the prescription will be waiting for you or you will take a paper prescription to the pharmacist and have it filled, just as you would a prescription from your own physician.

Mail-order catalogs, grocery, feed, pet-supply stores, and home-veterinary-care books also carry or describe a variety of over-the-counter (OTC), "natural" or "holistic" preparations. I strongly caution you against their use without first consulting your veterinarian.

Following Directions

It is especially important not to use any drugs, whether they are veterinary or human preparations, in a manner inconsistent with the directions on the label unless your veterinarian tells you specifically to do this. Cats metabolize many drugs very slowly and can easily be overdosed if they are given too much of a drug or are given the drug too often. Aspirin is one good example. Even the common anti-diarrhea medication Pepto-Bismol contains an aspirin-like ingredient.

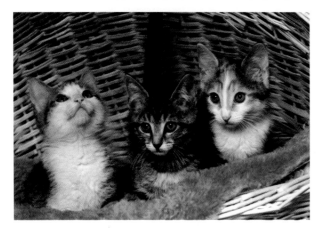

These drugs can be used safely in cats, but only with careful dosing. There are many, many drugs with routine extra-label uses in veterinary medicine, but they should be closely supervised. Acetaminophen (Tylenol, etc.), and ibuprofen (Advil, Motrin, etc.) are extremely toxic and should never be given to cats.

The amount of drug that is prescribed is based on your cat's weight, or for some medications, its body surface area. Your veterinarian also considers your cat's age or if it is pregnant. Kittens do not handle drugs as well as adult cats do, and we know that that is not very well indeed. Some drugs affect the developing skeleton, teeth, or nervous system. This could cause birth defects in the unborn fetus, or abnormal growth in young kittens. Your veterinarian will also consider any underlying diseases involving the kidney and liver, two organ systems important in metabolizing and eliminating drugs from the body. The goal is to achieve maximum benefit with minimal risk of toxicity.

It is very important that you follow the prescription directions and give your cat its medication on time and for the full duration of treatment. Be sure that you clearly understand the directions for use before you leave the office, including potential side effects, whether the medication needs to be kept in the refrigerator, and if it should be diluted, mixed, or shaken. Ask your veterinarian or veterinary technician these questions, as most pharmacists are not familiar with all the ins and outs of the drugs used for animals. Use a calendar (see page 39), to help you keep track of when and for how long you give each medication. If you keep a logbook or record of your pet's illnesses, write down the name and dosage of the drugs that were used to treat her, or peel off the label from the bottle or vial and stick it on the page. This is particularly useful if you have several pets. Over the years, it becomes difficult to recall just who had what problem and when!

Failure to complete a course of treatment can result in a relapse or, in the case of antibiotics, in the growth of bacteria resistant to the drug. My heart sinks when a client brings me a plastic bag full of assorted bottles and vials of old medicines, and uncompleted prescriptions saved "just in case she gets it again." They have invariably expired and lost their potency.

Your veterinarian has prescribed a course of therapy for your cat based on physical examination, appropriate laboratory tests, and experience. If your schedule limits your ability to give medication at certain times or if you find it easier to give your cat liquids versus pills, etc., let your veterinarian know this. She may be able to choose an equally effective preparation to accommodate your situation. Most treatments involve more than drugs; they involve rest, good nutrition, physical therapy and T.L.C.!

How to Give Medications

Yesterday, I noticed that my cat Willie has another eye infection. She gets these bouts of conjunctivitis about twice a year and although I open the cupboard where my veterinary supplies are stored at least once a day, somehow she knows that this time I will reach for a little tube of the ointment that I use to treat these infections. I turn around, and she has vanished.

Cocoa is no more cooperative than his housemate, though he'll stand his ground. Under no circumstances can I give that cat a pill or a dropperful of medicine by myself. I have a bag of clothes-turned-into-dustcloths from those lessons learned. Now I enlist the aid of a friend, or give the cat shots.

If you are facing a showdown with your own cat at this moment, this is a very good time to read "Achieving Cooperation" (see page 29).

Don't give your cat much time to figure out what's about to happen. Have the medication out of the bottle and ready so that you're not fumbling with the cap and the cat. Then fetch the patient.

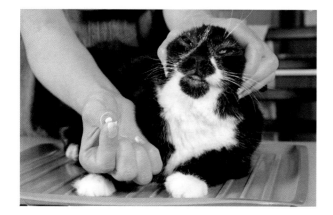

Tablets and Capsules

Medicine in the form of tablets or pills, capsules, and liquids are given by mouth. Once inside your cat, they dissolve in the stomach or somewhere along the intestinal tract. Some of the drug is absorbed into your cat's circulatory system, which then delivers it into the body tissues. Some of the drug never gets absorbed at all, and leaves with the feces. All body tissues do not take in the same amount of any particular drug flowing along with the blood. In fact, some tissues, such as the brain and the eye, have very effective barriers against chemicals. That's one reason why one antibiotic, for example, may be more useful than another, depending upon what tissue is infected.

If all that sounds very complicated, it is. It's important for you to know something of what happens to drugs once they are inside your cat, so that you can appreciate why it is important to give your cat his or her medicine on time and *finish the prescription*. So have your veterinarian or technician show you how to do this, give the medication, and follow these instructions if you need help.

I recommend that you work at a surface height about waist-high rather than bending or squatting over your cat on the floor. Some people find it easier to sit cross-legged and tuck their cat in. Depending on the cat, this is how a lot of clothes become dustcloths if Ripper decides to launch himself off your lap. Either way, position your cat with his back toward you, so that he can't back up. If you are right-handed, hold his head gently in your left hand, grasping just below the ears. With the pill or capsule in your right hand between your thumb and third finger, push his lower jaw down with your index finger and open the mouth. Place or drop the pill as far back on the tongue as you can. If you can give the pill a little nudge with your finger so that it goes over the base of the tongue, that helps to prevent him from working it forward and spitting it out. Quickly close his mouth and hold it shut. Stroke under the chin until he swallows the tablet.

Cats can be very clever, holding pills in their mouth, only to spit them out when your back is turned! More than one of my clients has assured me that their cat "got all the pills except the ones I found behind the couch..." Butter, peanut butter, petrolatum, or hairball laxatives will help hold the tablet to the roof of the mouth until your cat obliges you and swallows it. And if you're squeamish about sticking your fingers between your cat's teeth, there are wand-type devices that hold the pill for you. Once inserted over the back of his tongue, push the plunger to release the tablet.

Liquids and Pastes

Liquid medicines come either in the form of a *solution* or a *suspension*. Solutions are drugs dissolved

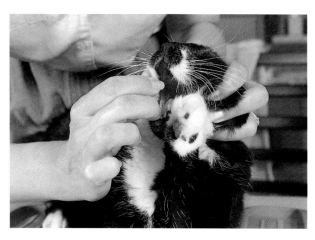

in water and are usually clear. Suspensions are cloudy mixtures of a drug powder in water. The particles of powder tend to settle out as the bottle sits undisturbed. Most veterinary hospitals and pharmacies will add the appropriate amount of water to a bottle of powdered drug for you. If you are doing this yourself, be sure that you measure and add exactly the right amount of water. Too much or too little water will result in the wrong concentration of drug in the suspension. This means that your cat will be under- or overdosed with the drug when you administer it. Drug suspensions usually require refrigeration and shaking prior to use.

Drug pastes are not as common, but they are basically the same as drug suspensions except that the powder is mixed with a thick, inert substance. Now the powder doesn't settle out in the tube as it does in water, so you don't have to shake it. In theory, pastes should

Use your third finger to pry open the lower jaw. Working on the kitchen table, presumably a surface upon which he's not allowed, will put him off guard for a few seconds giving you the advantage.

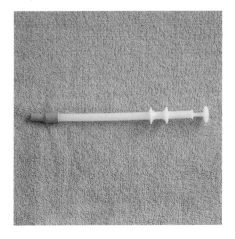

*Liquid med-
ication can
be adminis-
tered by
syringe or
dropper.
Be sure to
set the open
container of
medication
well out of
reach to pre-
vent it from
spilling if
your cat
scrambles
to get away.*

be easier to give than liquids because they stick to the inside of the mouth until your cat swallows it.

Liquids and pastes are administered with an eye dropper or an extension called a *catheter tip* on the tube. They have the advantage that you don't have to put your fingers into the cat's mouth. You also don't have to open his mouth as far, which is an important consideration for our less cooperative patients and for painful mouth conditions like severe periodontal disease or jaw fractures. One disad-

vantage is that medicines are not very palatable and unless you can squirt it way over the base of the tongue, your cat is going to get a not-so-pleasant-tasting mouthful.

To give liquids or pastes, hold his head gently below the ears as you would for pills or capsules. Insert the tip of the eye dropper or catheter between the teeth on the upper and lower jaw on the side of the cat's mouth. Some cats are more accepting of having the dropper or tip inserted from the front, between the incisors. Either approach will usually make cats open their mouth and make pushing motions with the tongue to get that thing out of there! Squirt the contents over the back of the tongue. It may take several squeezes of the bulb or plunger to do this thoroughly. Your cat might tolerate this better if you squirt small amounts into his mouth and allow him to swallow small portions of the dose at a time.

Until you get proficient at this, some of the medicine will be flung about if he shakes his head and tries to spit it out. If a large proportion of the dose is lost this way, your cat won't get enough of the medicine to be effective. If the medication comes in more than one form, switch to one that affords you greater success.

Adding medicine to the food is generally not an acceptable method of medicating your cat. The off-odor and flavor can be enough to make him refuse the meal or, owing to the "snacking" nature of a cat's appetite, the dose will be inadequate. Occasionally you can use this technique successfully if you add small quantities of medicine (a crushed pill) to absolutely very favorite foods. Try a tiny amount of unadulterated food the first time. If he eats it, mix the medication in the smallest amount he will eat at one time.

Eye Drops and Ointments

One summer, while living in a tiny apartment, I was slicing onions for a large batch of bread-and-butter pickles. Glancing over at my cats, I saw that tears were streaming down all our faces from the overwhelming onions! The eye is bathed in tears produced by glands located in the lids and in the tissues surrounding the eyeball itself. When an animal blinks, the eyelids sweep across the cornea like a squeegee. Tears collect and flow into tiny openings located in the corner of the eye. From there, tears flow into ducts running through the nose and are swallowed. If the eyes are irritated by chemicals, dust, allergies, or infection, more tears are produced than can drain away and be swallowed. In that case, the eyes and nose become "runny." That's why your nose runs when you cry, peel onions, or go out on a cold, windy day!

Most domestic animals also have a third eyelid called a *nictitating membrane*. If the eyes are irritated, this eyelid comes up and over the cornea more than usual. Sometimes this happens during general illness, unrelated to the eyes. Cats have some voluntary control over their third eyelid, meaning they can pull them up on their own, usually when they don't want their doctor to examine them!

This elaborate irrigation system explains why it is necessary to administer eye medication so frequently. The contact time for the medicine is actually very short, about 20 minutes, so the active ingredient must be absorbed into the eye tissues quickly. Many medications do not penetrate into the eye very effectively. For severe problems, we often use a combination of oral medication and topical ones. Because the consequences of eye problems are so devastating, it is especially important to give these medications timely and properly. If you have trouble doing so, consider hospitalizing your cat for treatment.

Avoid touching the catheter tip of the tube to any of the tissues around the eye as you instill a small strip of medication along the conjunctiva; or as ophthalmologists like to say about eye drops, "Bomb from above!"

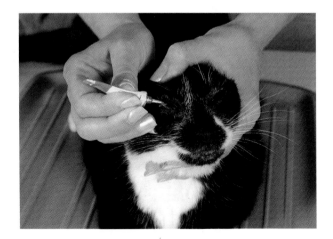

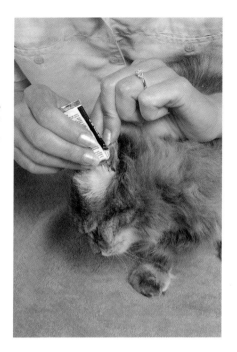

Pain and itching can make administering ear medications difficult. If there are ulcers near the opening, these may need to be treated and to heal before you can insert the catheter tip past these painful areas. This extends the length of the treatment period but is easier for your cat.

To instill eye drops or ointments, restrain your cat as you would for any oral medication. If your cat is very sensitive to having his eyes manipulated, you may need to scruff him or wrap him in a towel. Holding his head in your hand and tipping his nose upward will cause him to open his eyes wide enough to drop in the medication. If not, gently part the lids with your thumb and forefinger. For eye ointments, roll down his lower lid and squirt a small strip of ointment in the pocket. Gently open and close the lids to distribute the medication over the eye itself. To prevent contamination with bacteria, don't touch the tip of the container to the tissues surrounding the eye.

The third eyelid is sometimes used as a natural bandage to cover the cornea in cases of deep ulceration or laceration. Your veterinarian will use this technique by placing one or two temporary sutures in the margin of the lid and pulling it up over the cornea. The sutures are tied over a button or piece of rubber tubing that prevents them from cutting into the upper eyelid. This doesn't sound very pleasant, but it is very effective in protecting the damaged cornea and seems to reduce the pain. In these special cases, a small opening is left where the tip of an ointment tube can be inserted and medication instilled behind the closed lids.

Ear Drops and Ointments

The ear canals of domestic animals are shaped like the capital letter "L." There is a vertical portion that you can see, and a horizontal one that your veterinarian examines with an instrument called an *otoscope*. The eardrum is at the base of the canal at the end of the L. Drainage and air circulation for the ear canal is quite poor because of this anatomy. Ear infections tend to persist and recur. Medications must be dropped carefully into the opening, or a tube with a longer applicator tip must be used in order for the medicine to reach the horizontal portion of the canal.

To instill drops or ointments, grasp the ear flap gently with your thumb and forefinger and find the opening among all the nooks and crannies. Hold the tip of the dropper close to the opening and squeeze out the desired number of drops. For ointments, insert the tip of the tube straight down into the opening of the vertical canal and give a squeeze. Without letting go of the ear flap, gently massage below the ear so the medicine flows downward. Once you release your cat, he will shake his head and some of the medication will be flung back out onto you! The goal here is to get more in than is flung out.

Injections

The use of injectable medications is usually limited to the patients in the hospital. Proper dosing and administration of injections, or shots, requires quite a bit of expertise and manual dexterity, along with a proficiency in animal handling. Injectable medications are used most often for animals that are very ill and require frequent assessment by the attending veterinarian. Many state laws, not to mention common sense, require strict methods for disposal of syringes and needles.

There are a few notable exceptions to the in-hospital-only rule for injectable medicines, such as the administration of insulin to a diabetic cat. Cats like my cat Cocoa are another. It is impossible for one person to give that cat oral medications. For the few patients like him I have come across, it is much easier for their owners to give shots.

Injectable medication is given in one of three ways: *subcutaneously*, or under the skin, *intramuscularly*, or in the muscle, and *intravenously*, or in a vein or in IV fluids. There are a few others, but they are beyond the scope of this text. Subcutaneous (SQ) injections are the easiest and most frequently used. Properly done, they are nearly painless. Cats are endowed with a most advantageous physical trait, the loose skin over much of their bodies, especially between the shoulder blades. This is the location where most subcutaneous injections are given and where small pockets of fluids are often administered.

Syringes and needles come in a variety of sizes. Your veterinarian will provide you with the appropriate size for each. Do not use any other size syringe or needle than what you are shown; this could result in a serious under- or overdose of medication. To load a syringe with the proper dose, first "break the seal" by moving the plunger back and forth a few times. This will make it easier to draw up the dose. If the medication needs mixing, do this now. *If you are working with insulin, remember that this drug is very fragile. Mix insulin by gently rolling the bottle between your hands until it is uniformly in suspension.*

Insert the needle straight into the rubber stopper on the bottle. Hold the bottle with the syringe upside down against the palm of your hand. Make sure that the needle is inside the liquid, not above it, or you will draw in only air. Pull back the plunger, drawing the drug into the syringe beyond the amount that you wish to give. Release the plunger and tap on the barrel of the syringe to cause any air bubbles to rise and collect in a pocket just under the needle. Now push the plunger forward, pushing any air out through the needle, until the desired amount of the drug remains in the syringe. Remove the needle and replace the cap. Your veterinarian or veterinary technician should go through this procedure with you until you are thoroughly familiar with each step.

As with any other medication, have your syringe ready and the dose drawn before you even approach your cat. You may place your cat on a suitable waist-level

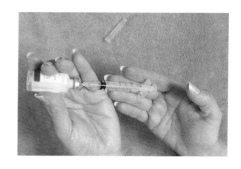

surface as usual, or sometimes I will suggest giving the injection while the cat is distracted by a plate of food. Either way, grasp the loose skin between the shoulder blades with your thumb and middle finger. Gently pull it upward to create a "tent." Feel for this with the forefinger of your other hand. Now, hold the syringe in your hand like a dart. Avoid the temptation to hold it with your thumb on the plunger. Only television doctors hold a syringe like that! Insert the needle into the tent. Pull back on the plunger and watch for a stream of blood to appear in the syringe. If there is, you have accidentally entered a blood vessel and you should withdraw the needle and try again. *Some injectable medications should not be given intravenously.* If no blood appears, push the plunger in all the way. Withdraw the needle.

To swab with alcohol or not to swab, that is always the question. Doctors and nurses almost always do. This does very little to disinfect the skin or fur, but wetting the fur does help to locate your "target."

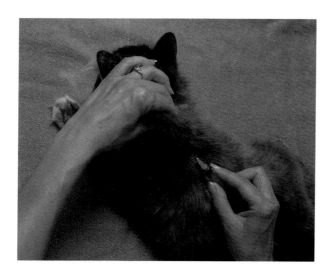

Naturally, you should not inject into an area that is grossly soiled with mud or dirt.

Subcutaneous Fluids

"Fluids," i.e., lactated Ringers, Ringers, dextrose, or sodium chloride solutions, are all clear, colorless liquids and contain a specific amount of salts and sugar that are "balanced" with the amount of the same substances in the blood. They are nonirritating to tissues and can be given subcutaneously or intravenously.

Subcutaneous administration can provide a cat with a reasonably large amount of fluid over a day's time. Your veterinarian may prescribe periodic fluids for a very old cat with kidney disease, who is drinking marginally enough water to meet his needs. Cats requiring long-term convalescent care for poisoning, liver disease, or trauma may be given fluids as a part of the overall therapy. There is a limit to the amount of fluid that a cat is capable of absorbing. The cat's need for fluid may exceed his capacity to absorb it from the subcutaneous tissues, and intravenous fluids will be necessary. Absorption will be influenced by your cat's body temperature. *Cats with a low body temperature cannot absorb subcutaneous fluids.*

Intravenous administration is a much more controlled and effective method of giving fluids to animals that are dehydrated, need circulatory support, or large volumes of fluid.

Intravenous fluids require that a catheter be inserted into a vein. A number of veins are located close enough to the surface of the skin to be useful for this purpose: on the foreleg, on the inside of the thigh, on the outside of the ankle, and on the neck. These veins collapse easily when an animal shifts its position or draws back a limb. Many veterinarians use a pump to accurately control the rate of intravenous flow and prevent the patient from receiving too much or too little fluid. There are some creative bandaging techniques that also help. I am explaining these things, not because intravenous fluids will be used very often in the home, but because you may see your cat trussed up in one of these devices in the hospital, and that can be very upsetting if you don't understand why.

Fluids come in glass bottles or plastic bags and are usually dispensed in the one-liter size, about one quart. The container is calibrated in 20-milliliter increments on the side. A milliliter is a metric unit of measure. There are about five

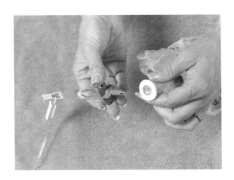

Insert the spiked drip chamber into the hole in the fluid bag.

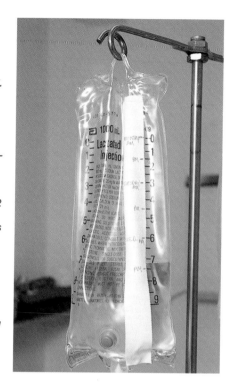

milliliters in one teaspoon. The amount of liquid in the bottle can be read when it is either right side up or when it is hung upside down by its plastic handle. One end of an IV set has a drip chamber so you can see the fluid flow. This end plugs into a rubber or plastic stopper in the container. The other end is fitted with a needle.

Most IV-set packages have illustrated instructions on the back showing how to assemble a fluid set-up, and your veterinary technician should show you how to do it the first time too. First unwrap the IV line. There will be a protective cap on the spiked end of the drip

chamber. This apparatus is sterile, so don't remove the cap or touch it to any surface until you insert it into the bag or bottle. Next, peel off the metal tab and remove the metal cap over the end of the glass bottle to expose the sterile rubber stopper. Force the spike into the rubber stopper. If you are working with a plastic bag, peel off the plastic tab. Notice that there is a large hole, so don't turn the bag upside down until you have inserted the spiked end of the IV set.

Turn the bag or bottle upside down. Squeeze the drip chamber to create a slight vacuum, drawing fluid into the chamber up to the line. The apparatus can be suspended from a shower curtain or kitchen cabinet handle. Gravity causes the fluid to run through the line. Remove the protective cap from the end of the line and run out any air. Replace the cap with the appropriate size needle. There is a clamping device on the line to stop the flow. Air accidentally injected subcutaneously is not harmful to your cat.

Place your cat on the work surface and lift the loose skin between his shoulder blades to form a tent, as you would to give any subcutaneous injection. Insert the needle into the center of the tent. Your cat will feel very little discomfort. Roll open the clamp on the IV line and pinch it open if the plastic tube remains flattened. A steady stream of liquid should run into the drip chamber. If it flows too slowly, rotate the needle under the skin until a steady stream forms.

Note the level of fluid at the start, and where the level should be when the proper dose has been given. I put a piece of adhesive tape along the calibration marks, and mark with a pen where each dose should start and stop. There will probably be little need to restrain your cat other than to scratch his ears and chin. He may shift around a bit as the pocket of fluid forms. The stretching this causes may be slightly uncomfortable, in which case you should create several small pockets rather than one large one. Pinch the skin where the needle exits as you withdraw the needle. A few drops of fluid might leak back out of the hole. Sometimes this is slightly blood-tinged, but this is normal. Place the cap back on the needle. The same needle can be used for two or three doses of fluid *on the same animal.*

The fluid will be absorbed over several hours. Gravity will cause it to flow downward and your cat may develop very saggy elbows! If any significant fluid remains at the time of the next dose, you should contact your veterinarian. Your cat may be unable to absorb the necessary dose and intravenous fluids may be required.

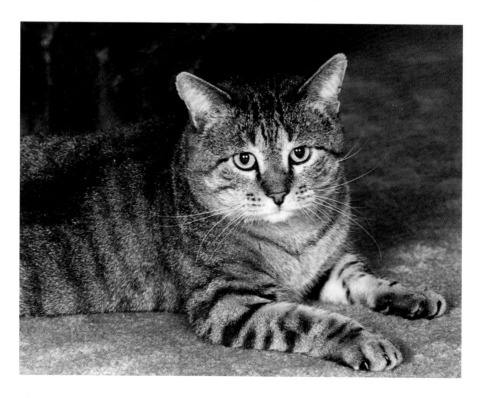

Chapter 10
Basic Nursing

Compressing Wounds and Injuries

Compressing is one of the oldest and most universally practiced forms of medicine. Historically, it has involved the application of heat or cold, and sometimes salts, solutions, herbs, poultices, or other medicaments by way of cloth pads to the surface of the skin. The effectiveness of these substances has been judged largely on the basis of folklore and time-honored home remedies rather than on scientific fact. However, contemporary medicine does use compressing and in its simplest form, it provides excellent relief from pain and infection and promotes rapid wound healing.

Hot compressing is employed in the treatment of infected wounds. It stimulates blood flow to the affected area, bringing in antibiotics, antiinflammatory and analgesic medications through the circulation. Compressing promotes drainage of infected wounds. The warmth alone often provides excellent pain relief. Many cats will recognize this particular benefit after the first application and will relax and seem to enjoy the experience. Moist hot compresses clean the wound. Epsom salts and antiseptics added to the compressing solutions in appropriate amounts can inhibit infection and encourage rapid wound healing.

Before you compress your cat's wound, have everything you need assembled and ready to use. Pure warm water directly from the faucet or in a pan is entirely adequate; however, some veterinarians add a small but specific amount of surgical solution or epsom salts added to the warm tap water. Occasionally the doctor may want you to use a sterile prepared solution. In this case, warm the solution for a few (3 to 4) seconds in a microwave oven or in a pan of hot water. Use a soft, clean cloth such as a face cloth or short stack of gauze sponges. My personal favorite is squares cut from cloth diapers, because they are thick, soft, highly absorbent, and can be laundered and re-used. The cloth should be wet but not dripping and should be as warm as can be comfortably tolerated.

Remember that inflamed, injured tissue is more sensitive to heat than your hands and can scald easily.

I like to do this procedure next to a sink because I have more control over the cat while working at waist level and I like to take advantage of the running water to rinse out the cloth thoroughly. Not every cat tolerates the sound of running water. You may find this task most easily accomplished by holding your cat on your lap. Hold the damp cloth on the wound for about 10 minutes. Rinse the cloth as often as necessary to keep it warm and clean. When you pull the cloth away from the wound, the surface debris will stick to the cloth and be removed.

Dry, hot compressing can give the same benefits as hot moist compressing—increased circulation and pain relief—if you place a warm, wet cloth inside a plastic bag before applying it to the skin. This technique is sometimes used to reduce the swelling associated with surgical incisions, which should always remain dry.

Cold compressing is used within the first hour of a traumatic orthopedic injury to reduce swelling. It can also be very effective in controlling bleeding. Except in an emergency, cold compression should not be used without the recommendation of a veterinarian. Put some crushed ice in a small plastic bag and then wrap it in several layers of toweling to prevent freezing the skin. Gently place the compress on the affected part.

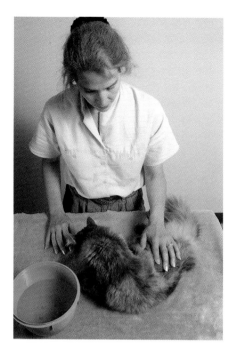

Despite the fact that water is involved, many cats seem to enjoy the hot compressing. If she won't cooperate at first, give her something to eat during the treatment as we did here with Carly. If that fails, have an assistant scruff or stretch her.

Repeat as recommended by your veterinarian.

Flushing Wounds

The practice of wound flushing is controversial. Some doctors believe that the solutions used for flushing are toxic to tissues and will delay wound healing. By flushing wounds, you could also introduce other germs into the wound and set up the possibility of a more severe and persistent infection. Flushing wounds can help to rinse pus and debris from an area while instilling an antiseptic solution that kills bacteria. Saline (salt) water, peroxide, and a variety of surgical antiseptics are commonly used for this purpose. Saline has the advantage of being nontoxic; however it has little germ-killing ability. Peroxide has a great visual effect and mechanically removes pus and debris, but it is very toxic to tissues and should be used only when diluted and on the recommendation of your veterinarian.

Surgical solutions such as povidone-iodine (Betadine) or chlorhexidine diacetate (Nolvasan) kill a broad spectrum of germs; however, povidone-iodine is not an effective antiseptic in the presence of blood and pus. When used, povidone-iodine should be diluted to the color of weak tea. Chlorhexidine diacetate should be diluted to 0.75 percent. Follow your veterinarian's instructions for diluting the flush solutions. *Full-strength Betadine and other povidone-iodine solutions are less effective than dilute ones; both are toxic to living tissues unless properly diluted.*

Your veterinarian will provide you with the appropriate flushing solution and syringe if she feels it is a necessary part of wound management. Be sure to keep any diluting containers and syringes scrupulously clean with hot soap water and rinse them well. Store these supplies in a clean, dry place. Wash your hands thoroughly before and after the procedure.

To flush an open wound properly, use a large volume of appropriately diluted solution and a high jet pressure from the syringe. Expect the solution to splatter as you force the solution through the syringe as quickly as possible. The jet pressure acts to lift debris and bacteria off the surface of the wound. This is more effective, less damaging, and less painful than merely wiping the surface with gauze.

An abscess is a pocket of pus and damaged tissue under the skin. It develops as a result of puncture wounds, usually from the bite of another cat. Abscesses usually rupture and drain to the outside through a small opening. Sometimes they become progressively larger, undermining large areas of skin. Abscesses tend to drain very poorly unless they rupture through a large opening or are lanced. It is often necessary to place one or more drains through the abscess. Drains are usually of several types: soft rubber Penrose drains, antibiotic impregnated gauze, or cloth drains called umbilical tape. The latter two look a lot like shoe laces tied through the skin! Penrose drains are usually sutured in place.

Drains permit the accumulation of pus and other debris to flow to the exterior from pockets under the skin and thus allow healing. Without good drainage, infections tend to fester and recur.

The solution used for flushing closed wounds should be at or slightly warmer than body temperature. When flushing wounds with drains, the syringe is filled and the tip inserted under the skin where the drain exits. The contents of the syringe are squirted under the skin and into the pocket. The flushing solution will run out the openings in the skin, bringing with it pus and sloughing tissue. This process is repeated several times until the solution becomes clear. *Note that you do not flush solutions through the center of a Penrose drain as they do not have holes.* The drains themselves are removed by your veterinarian after two or three days.

The exact volume of flushing solution used is not important. These solutions should be slightly warm to the touch. Remember that damaged tissue is much more sensitive to burns.

Therapeutic Baths

Because most cats have a natural aversion to water, you will probably need assistance in giving your cat a bath—one person to hold the slippery creature and one person to lather and rinse. Before beginning, insert a piece of cotton into each ear canal to absorb the water that will inevitably get inside. Instill a small amount of neutral eye ointment (get this from your veterinarian) into both eyes to protect them from soapy run-off. The best place to give a bath at home is in the kitchen sink where you will be working at waist level in a good size basin. Have a couple of clean bath

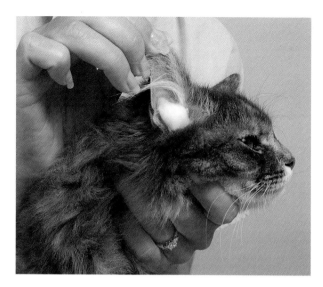

towels ready for your wet feline when it's all over.

Follow the instructions on the shampoo or other solution unless otherwise instructed by your veterinarian. Most medicated and insecticidal shampoos require contact with the skin and coat for several minutes for maximum benefit, so watch the clock. Use a face cloth to rinse around the head to help prevent soap from getting into the eyes. To rinse, use a small saucepan, bowl, or sprayer attachment on the sink. Spend a lot of time rinsing, and pay close attention to rinsing under the legs and tummy where soap tends to collect. Soap residues are one of the most common causes of skin irritations. The medicated and insecticidal shampoos dispensed by your veterinarian are formulated to be extremely rinsable, and are superior to over-the-counter preparations.

Before a bath, put some cotton in your cat's ears. After a bath, clean them with a little rubbing alcohol to remove any water left in the ear canals.

When rinsing is complete, dry your cat thoroughly, using several towels and a blow dryer if your cat will tolerate it. A soft wire brush called a slicker brush will remove the loose hair. Remember that inflamed skin is very sensitive to heat and cold and your cat can be more easily burned by bath water or a dryer.

Enemas

As some cats get older, they lose the ability to empty their bowels effectively. Such cats are more than constipated, they are obstipated. Impacted feces causes severe distension of the colon. These cats are in pain and seriously ill. The condition is managed in a variety of ways, including manipulating the amount of fiber in the diet, laxatives, regularly scheduled enemas, and sometimes surgery. Never give your cat an enema unless your veterinarian has instructed you to do so, and only after she demonstrates the procedure.

You need two people to give an enema properly and safely. Your veterinarian will provide you with an enema solution specifically made for animals, or you may be instructed to use a home "recipe" with warm water and an empty human enema bottle such as a Fleets. Under no circumstances should you use a human enema solution in a cat. They are very high in phospho-

rus and are extremely toxic to cats.

Let's be forthright here—this is not a pleasant process, and most people recognize that a veterinary hospital is usually better equipped to manage giving an enema and its aftereffects. Still, if you need to take care of this at home, I suggest that you work in the bathtub. One person should restrain your cat by holding onto the scruff. The person working at the other end of the cat should lubricate the catheter tip of the enema bottle with a small amount of petroleum jelly or K-Y jelly and gently insert it into the rectum as you would a thermometer. Insert the catheter tip to its fullest extent. If you cannot because of fecal impaction, contact your veterinarian. Slowly and gently express the contents of the enema bottle into the colon and withdraw the nozzle. It's a good idea to have a litterbox right there by the tub, as most cats head right for it. If you have a large dog crate, put your cat in there with the box. It may take 30 minutes or so before you see results.

Cleaning Eyes and Nose

Remove the crusty debris that accumulates around the eyes of cats and kittens with upper respiratory infections with a soft cotton ball and either boric acid eyewash or a sterile, preservative-free (aerosol spray) saline solution made for soft contact lenses. You and your cat should not use the same bottle of saline to prevent one of you from giving the other an eye infection! I prefer using saline solutions to plain tap water because the latter is not balanced and can be irritating. Do not spray saline directly into your cat's eyes.

Use a very wet cotton pad or soft cloth to clean your cat's nose of mucus and crusts that accumulate with respiratory infections. For very heavily dried-on debris, soften the crust by applying a small amount of antibiotic ointment, K-Y, or petroleum jelly, and wait a few minutes before wiping it off. Repeat as often as you need to keep the nose clean, since your cat won't eat if she can't smell food.

Cleaning and Flushing Ears

Before you clean your cat's ears, see page 74 for information on giving ear drops and ointments so that you are familiar with the anatomy of the ear. Your cat's ear canals are proportionately longer than your own and are L-shaped, angling inward. The horizontal portion of the canal tends to accumulate debris and pus if it is infected. Therefore, medications put into the ear may be ineffective unless these materials are periodically removed.

Your veterinarian will provide you with an appropriate ear-cleaning solution. The solution will either be pre-mixed, or you will need to mix it yourself in a small bowl; you will also need a small bulb or ear cleaning syringe from the drugstore. You will also need some cotton, a small towel, and a few cotton swabs. If the ears are very sore and itchy, you will probably need an assistant.

Working at waist level on a good solid surface as you are now accustomed to doing, hold the tip of your cat's ear and examine the opening to the ear canal. Using the squirt bottle or bulb syringe, instill sufficient solution to fill and overfill the ear canal so that the solution spills back out of the ear. This is going to tickle your cat and you, as the solution trickles down her neck and probably your sleeve. While still holding onto the ear, gently massage the base of the canal to break up debris, working it upwards towards the opening. Your cat will find this less objectionable if the solution is slightly warm. Besides the tickling, the sound of the ear canal being filled and the squishing sound as you massage annoys your cat the most.

Using several pieces of cotton and your finger, wipe out the ear. You can use cotton swabs in the nooks and crannies, but do not insert them into the canal. This serves only to pack debris into the base. Repeat the process until the cotton stays reasonably clean. Then medicate the ear as directed.

Brushing Your Cat's Teeth

Good oral hygiene may sound ridiculous to you. I have seen eyes roll and heard the argument: "Wild cats never brush their teeth and they do just fine!" In nature, a cat's diet consists of whole, small animals. Crunching on little bones serves to scrape the teeth and keep them healthy. Feral cats die at a younger age from infectious diseases and accidents, and therefore don't live long enough to develop the severe dental problems seen so frequently in well-cared for housecats. With modern vaccines, improved nutrition, and regular health care, it is not unusual for a cat to live 15 to 20 years, much longer than the cats we may have grown up with. And that is ample time to develop cavities and severe periodontal disease.

Your cat can sit up or lie down to have her teeth brushed. Carly prefers to recline.

In fact, cavities are extremely common in cats and can cause a great deal of low-grade mouth pain that goes unnoticed by an owner, until those teeth are loose and decayed. Once a process destructive to the periodontal ligament that holds the teeth in the jaw begins, it continues until the teeth loosen, fracture, and fall out. As in humans, some cats develop tooth and gum problems more readily than others. When the cavities are filled and the diseased teeth are removed, the cat returns to eating normally and owners tell me, "She's acting like a kitten again."

There are also some viral diseases and immune system diseases that can result in chronic gingivitis and periodontal disease. Your veterinarian examines your cat's mouth during her annual physical examination, assesses the need for professional scaling and polishing, and gives you pointers on home care. *Your home care will only be effective after your cat's teeth have been professionally cleaned and any existing infection is under control.*

Use a cotton swab, small child's toothbrush, or a specially manufactured pet toothbrush to brush your cat's teeth. I find that the cotton swab is the least objectionable to the cat. Moisten the swab or brush with a veterinary dentifrice, peroxide, water from a water-packed can of tuna, or an oral antiseptic prepared for animals. Do not use

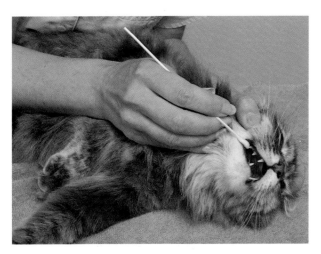

human toothpaste or mouthwash as they may burn or upset your cat's stomach, if swallowed.

Moisten the swab and then go find your cat. Cats seem to know what you're up to and immediately vanish. Put her on the kitchen table facing away from you so she can't back up. Hold her head in your hand as you would to give her a pill. You don't need to open her mouth, just slide the swab into the corner and gently rub the teeth and gums along the back, sides, and front. You do not need to brush the inside or occlusive (grinding) surfaces of the teeth.

With a little practice, the whole process takes about 30 seconds. Daily brushing is best; if this isn't possible, try for three times a week. To mimic the natural teeth cleaning action of the feral cat, offer your cat cooked chicken necks once or twice a week. She will crunch up these neck bones safely and scrape her teeth in the process. Cooking softens the bones and makes passage through the gastrointestinal tract safer. Do not feed other chicken bones, which may fragment into dangerous splinters. Do not feed raw chicken, which may cause salmonella food poisoning.

Not all cats will eat chicken necks. The best oral hygiene begins when a cat is still a young kitten. That way she becomes accustomed to having her teeth brushed. However, I have seen many older cats adapt to routine home care. And you can take comfort in the fact that I did not ask you to floss.

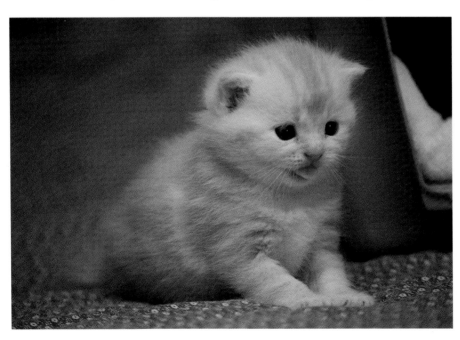

Chapter 11

Managing Bandages and Splints

Incisions

Convalescing cats with an incision should be confined indoors for a minimum of 7 to 10 days. This is to prevent the surgical wound from opening up or becoming contaminated with dirt or germs. The movement of skin at the incision site during ordinary activity can delay the healing process. That's why a wound under a foreleg takes so much longer to heal than one on the head, for example. Also, it would be very unfortunate if your cat were to catch a suture while creeping under the bushes or poking through fences and pull the wound open. So despite any protestations to the contrary, keep your cat indoors, at least until the stitches are removed. And afterwards, it's not a bad idea to continue the confinement for a few more days until the scar tissue matures, and the wound is less likely to be pulled open.

Although most cats are fairly tolerant of their incisions and leave them alone, a few cats will try to remove the sutures. I suspect that cats experience an itching sensation as the wound heals and the fur grows in, just like people. Be particularly vigilant if your cat has any type of drain. Your fastidious feline might be perturbed by the trickle of drainage, clean himself, and chew the drain out when you're not looking.

Elizabethan Collars

While dogs will often eat the drain, cats usually leave them lying around just to annoy you. Many cats remove the sutures in their toes on their own several days after a declawing procedure. This is seldom a problem. Don't expect any cat with a urethral catheter or sutures in the urogenital area not to lick and try to pull them out. These cats, or any others that you suspect may be a problem, should wear what is called an Elizabethan (E.) collar.

E. collars are funnel-like barriers that cover the head. They can snap around the neck or slip over the face. A piece of gauze or a regular cat collar is threaded through several loops and tied or fastened moderately snugly to prevent the cat from slipping the collar off. When slipping the collar over the head, avoid accidentally poking the cat's eyes with the loops.

E. collars are most effective when they extend just past the nose. Some cats manage to devise a way to scratch the incision with the edge of the collar. Most cats quickly learn how to eat with the collar in place. If you have to remove it at mealtime, be sure to put it back on as soon as your cat has finished eating. Alternatives to E. collars like aversion substances, such as bitter apple, pepper sauce, etc., are not always well tolerated by cats.

Appliances

Without exception, all cats sporting an E. collar, feeding tube, drain, bandage, cast, or splint should be confined indoors. Bandages, casts, and splints, sometimes called appliances, should be kept clean and dry. I once had a young feline patient with a broken foreleg, for which I applied a nice lightweight fiberglass cast. Three times. Every other day for one week, the owner brought his cat and its cast into the hospital in a box, although not attached to one another. Every other day for one week, I reapplied the cast and sent the cat home,

admonishing the owner to keep him indoors. "Somehow" the confinement would only last for half a day before he would escape and deposit the cast on the front stoop. I never did figure out how that cat got that cast off. Eventually the fracture healed, owing to the patient's youth, and the fact that we were dealing with a cat.

Fortunately, most cats tolerate appliances well. In fact, if your cat does fuss, there may be a problem with the appliance. Swelling of a bandaged limb causes the bandage to become tighter. Or, as the swelling goes down, it may have become loose and slipped out of position.

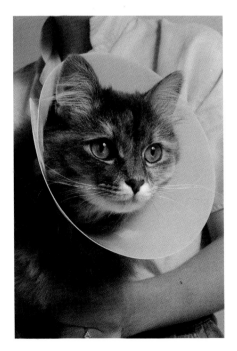

An Elizabethan collar.

Examine your cat's bandage or other appliance for wetness and positioning twice a day. Check the toes protruding from the dressing; they should be warm. Contact your veterinarian if you should detect pain, odor, or swelling associated with any appliance, or if they become wet or dirty. Examine the skin daily where bandage or cast material may be rubbing, such as under the foreleg for irritation and abrasion. There are serious consequences for complications associated with appliances that include extensive infection, tissue slough, or even loss of a limb.

Use a low-sided litterbox until your cat learns to maneuver efficiently with an appliance. Change the litterbox filler frequently, several times a day if necessary, to prevent the appliance from becoming soiled with feces or urine. Depending upon the type of bandage or casting material and how it is applied, you may need to use a different type of filler. The fine-grained clumping type gets between your cat's toes and into the bandage padding.

When a broken bone is set using a cast or a splint, it is essential that both the joint above and the joint below the fracture be immobilized. Failure to immobilize these joints will leave the fracture very unstable, and the cast could act as a lever, prying it open. Unstable fractures do not heal very well, even in cats.

Pins and wires are used to stabilize fractures that occur in bones above the knee or the elbow joints. This technique is called internal fixation. The broken bones are realigned and held together tightly without having to immobilize joints. Internal fixation lets the cat begin to use the broken leg much more quickly than with a cast or a splint. There are usually fewer complications and less chance of a permanant loss of function.

However, there are a few complications with the use of internal fixation. Metal pins begin to migrate and shift out of position during the healing process, especially if the patient is very active. They will take the path of least resistance, and can move into joints and even back themselves out of the bone. Sudden lameness or pain in an otherwise pain-free, recuperating cat suggests a problem with the pins. You may feel the tip of the pin under the skin or actually see it begin to protrude and create a small hole draining a clear, pinkish fluid. If you notice this, call your veterinarian.

A third but seldom used method of fracture repair is through the use of a brace made with pins that enter the bones through the skin, and are connected together on the outside with crossbars and clamps. Imagine a sort of Erector Set, or Tinker Toys attached to your cat. This is called a Kirschner-Ehmer (K-E) apparatus and it is particularly useful if there are a lot of small fragments to the fracture, where other forms of fixation would be technically impractical or impossible. A K-E apparatus can and does loosen over time, and can also fall off if the cat is too active. Naturally, cats with a K-E apparatus should never go outdoors, and as this is not a particularly aesthetic approach to fracture repair, you will probably not want your cat on display anyway. Your veterinarian will request that you bring your cat to the hospital to have the screws tightened and the pins checked regularly for loosening. Despite the fact that pins are protruding from the bone, infection is generally not a problem, although there will be some pinkish-yellow serum drainage from the skin.

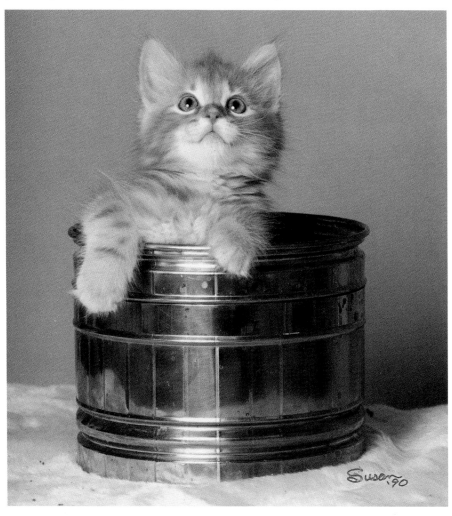

Chapter 12

Before and After Surgery and Dentistry

Preparing for Surgical and Dental Procedures

There are three classifications of surgical procedures: *elective*, such as neutering operations; *non-elective*, such as surgical biopsies; and *emergency* operations, such as those life-saving procedures that might be necessary if your cat is hit by a car. Depending upon the urgency of the surgery, there are several steps that you should take to prepare your cat and yourself for the procedure.

Let's assume that you are planning to have your six-month-old

Induction of anesthesia. This cat was first given a sedative by injection, and now a gas anesthetic is being delivered by mask. When the cat is completely asleep, Dr. Lasser will remove the mask and insert the blue and orange endotracheal tube (lower right corner of table) between the vocal cords and directly into the trachea.

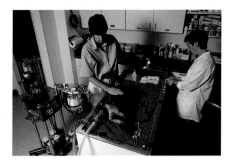

calico cat spayed next week. The night before the surgery, pick up your cat's bowl and withhold all food and treats after 6 PM. That means that if you have several cats, you'll need to confine her to a room of her own, or withhold food from all of them to prevent your patient from sneaking a snack. Most veterinarians agree that you can and should continue to leave water available at all times.

By withholding food for at least 12 hours before surgery, your cat's stomach is likely to be empty. One fairly common side effect of most anesthetics is nausea and vomiting. Postoperative vomiting can result in aspiration or inhalation of stomach contents into the lungs. A caustic mixture of food and stomach acids can cause a severe, often fatal pneumonia. If your cat does happen to be fed on the morning of surgery, be sure to inform your veterinarian. The surgery may proceed as planned, but she may be scheduled for later in the day to allow this meal to be digested.

Withholding food is important for all elective and nonelective procedures. Your veterinarian will take additional precautions to minimize the chance of vomiting and aspiration if emergency surgery is necessary. Because this forced fast is clearly a break in her normal routine, don't let your cat outside the next morning, as she may go off to find her own breakfast and will be indisposed when it's time to leave for the hospital.

The admitting staff member will ask you to sign a permission slip authorizing the anesthesia and procedure at the time of admission to the hospital. Ask for an estimate on the cost of the surgery, preferably in writing. Keep in mind that what you will receive is exactly that, an estimate. Because there is no way to know all the complications and findings at surgery beforehand even in routine elective surgery, the estimate may be different from the actual bill.

For example, your calico may be pregnant at the time of spaying. This condition adds to the surgery time and amount of supplies, and most veterinarians charge accordingly. The same holds true for biopsies, exploratories, fracture repairs, etc.

Ask your veterinarian or veterinary technician for some of the details of the surgery, for instance what exactly will be removed at the time of a neutering, where the incision will be, whether or not there will be any stitches, if they will have

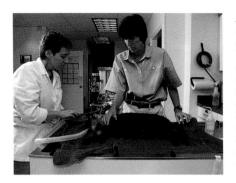

An endotracheal tube is now in place. These tubes allow for efficient and safe delivery of anesthetic gas to the patient and ensure an open airway for delivery of oxygen should there be complications under anesthesia. A veterinary technician will prepare the patient for surgery, monitor the patient's vital signs, and assist the doctor during the procedure.

to be removed and when. Learn how long your cat will be in the hospital and if there will be any special care or confinement necessary after she comes home. Ask about any medication or special diet. By finding out about these things ahead of time, you can begin to prepare early rather than at the time of discharge.

After Surgical and Dental Procedures

It takes anywhere from less than one hour to a day or more for the general anesthetics routinely used in veterinary practice to be completely eliminated from the body. Gas anesthetics, such as isofluorane, are rapidly eliminated; they are especially useful in very sick or old patients because of their high degree of safety. They are also useful in fractious patients who require anesthesia simply to allow the doctor to draw a blood sample. Combinations of injectable drugs have certain advantages that make them useful for some procedures. They are usually eliminated more slowly from the body, so your cat will recover more slowly as well.

Your cat's length of stay in the hospital will depend upon the nature of the illness and surgery, and the type of anesthetic that was required. Many people ask about watching the procedure while their cat is under anesthesia on the operating table or immediately post-op. Your veterinarian will have his own policy concerning observation. I caution against this as many owners who vow to remain stoic become weak-kneed at the sight of their own animal under anesthesia. And veterinarians have enough on their hands without catching the owner before they hit the floor.

Most veterinary hospitals also have a policy regarding visitation. Visitations are often permitted during specific hours, and *you should call ahead*. The nursing staff will probably welcome any offer you make to feed your cat and provide simple nursing care. Just check with them first before you feed him anything or move him out of his cage. He may have a special diet, get tangled in an IV line, be in more pain if lifted, or simply be too grouchy.

When it is time to go home, your veterinarian should provide you with instructions relating to your cat's care. This includes diet, exercise, degree of confinement, medication, and possible complications.

Don't be afraid to ask for details in writing if you think you can't remember it all. Ask for a demonstration of anything you are not certain you know how to do, such as how to give the medication. Find out who to call in case of an emergency after hours. You may be instructed to call an affiliated emergency clinic if there is a problem.

With few exceptions, you should assume that any cat with an incision should at the very least be confined indoors for 7 to 10 days. This applies to any incision, whether there are external sutures or not. See page 88 for a discussion of the specifics of confinement and adjusting to the return home.

When an animal is under anesthesia, the core body temperature drops because of the effects of the anesthetic on the circulatory system and the muscles. For several hours after waking, your cat may shiver. This is a normal physiologic response. The muscle trembling generates heat and raises your cat's temperature back to normal. Of course you can help by safely providing an external source of heat. I suggest your lap! Also keep in mind that if your cat's fur was clipped for an incision, he has lost important insulation against the cold air temperature and will be more susceptible to loss of body heat.

Another common question owners have is, "When should I feed my cat?" Because anesthetics can cause nausea and vomiting, and because his stomach has been empty for some time, feed your cat only a small portion of food, if anything at all, on the first night home. Except for a few specific instances, cats should not go more than 48 hours without food.

Here are some general things for you to watch for:

Anorexia or inappetence: We have already said that it is wise not to overfeed your cat soon after he has experienced an anesthetic. Most cats will eat at least one-quarter of their usual amount of food on the first day it is offered. If that stays down and if there is no specific reason to withhold food, you should increase the amount of food offered as quickly as possible, until your cat is back to eating his normal amount. This may occur as quickly as 24 hours post-anesthetic. If your cat does not show an interest in food within the first 24 to 36 hours, you should contact your veterinarian.

Cough: Gas anesthetic is delivered to the lungs by a tube placed between the vocal cords and into the trachea or windpipe. Placement of the tube and contact with these delicate tissues can cause a mild irritation, which in turn can cause him to cough. It should last only a day or two.

Dehiscence: The number one source of bacteria in a surgical infection is the patient himself. Your cat has bacteria that normally live on his skin and cause no harm. However, his immune system and his ability to fight infection is suppressed with the trauma and stress associated with surgery, allowing these bacteria to multiply, causing disease. Along with a discharge, infected tissues appear red, moist, and swollen and they may have a foul odor. The swelling causes the stitches to tighten and cut into the skin. The wound margins are no longer held together and begin to gap. This process is called "dehiscence" (pronounced: dee-hiss-ence). This infection can spread under the skin or into deeper tissues. Before it reaches those stages, call your veterinarian.

Depression: Your cat may be quieter than usual and spend most of his time sleeping until the anesthetic has been eliminated from the body. Discomfort and pain contribute to this. You should see a steady increase in the waking-time and an increase in normal behavior. You should be concerned if this does not progress as you expected, based on the recommendation of your veterinarian, or if your cat regresses.

Diarrhea: This is a fairly common occurrence after an anesthesia or surgical procedure and is probably a result of a number of factors, including the return to eating after the necessary fast, a change in diet, the stress associated with the procedure and hospitalization, antibiotics or other drugs, or from some kind of "bug" your cat may have picked up at the hospital. Diarrhea as a result of the first three factors will resolve uneventfully after two or three days.

Discharge and odor: It is perfectly normal for healing wounds to ooze a clear or pinkish-yellow, sticky fluid called *serum*. In areas where there is a lot of loose skin or movement, like under the foreleg, this fluid can accumulate in a pocket creating a *seroma*. Although seromas can resolve on their own, they often require a pressure bandage or drainage to prevent them from getting bigger. You should be concerned about any discharge other than serum. A white, yellow, or green discharge with foul odor means an infection has developed and you should call your veterinarian. If you can, check your cat's temperature before you call.

Fever: Because even the most delicate tissue handling results in inflammation, it is very common for patients to develop a slight fever of one or two degrees above normal for a day or two after surgery. A fever does not necessarily mean that an infection is present. Antibiotics may or may not be necessary.

Hemorrhage or bleeding: In small amounts, a drop or two of blood that oozes and collects at a place along the incision and then clots and dries is not a problem. This bleeding usually comes from a very small blood vessel in the skin that was stretched and started to bleed when your cat moved around. Continuous oozing or flow of any significance warrants a call to your veterinarian. It could mean that there is hemorrhage from a larger blood vessel that needs to be ligated or tied off to prevent significant blood loss. Bleeding from a vessel inside a body cavity is more difficult to detect. Internal bleeding into the abdomen may cause your cat's abdomen to become enlarged. Of course that would not occur with bleeding into the chest, as the rib cage does not allow the same expansion. Internal bleeding would most likely cause shocklike signs of pale gums and a rapid, weak pulse. See page 47 for details on monitoring these vital signs.

Swelling, heat, and redness: In moderation, these are normal and natural parts of the process of inflammation. Swelling represents an influx of fluid and components of the immune system that bind, heal, and repair. Aside from the trauma that the tissues sustain even from delicate and precision handling, the suture material used to close the incision also incites the inflammation response, particularly the "dissolvable" kinds. The swelling can be intense if a cat is sensitive to the type of suture material used.

Heat is given off as a result of the biochemical reactions involved in inflammation. This extra heat, along with the opening up of the blood supply into the area, causes a pink flush to the skin and the noticeable increase in skin temperature. Of course, this would only be noticeable in areas where the fur was shaved or naturally thin, like over the eyes. These signs in the absence of pain, odor, or discharge, will usually resolve on their own or with compressing.

Pain: It's very difficult to assess the amount of pain your cat is feeling. Being so stoic, cats don't often draw on the sympathies of their owners as do our canine counterparts. We extrapolate the potential for pain in many situations from ourselves. We also assess pain by our cat's appetite, activity level, desire for companionship, and even the look in their eyes! *The common painkillers used in dogs, aspirin and phenylbutazone, are extremely toxic to cats.* The only safe and effective drugs to control pain in cats are given by injection and must be used in the hospital and under the supervision of a veterinarian. Pain relief at home is best offered by rest, quiet, warmth, treatments like compressing, and antibiotics if appropriate. If you feel your cat is in unnecessary pain, call your veterinarian.

Pallor: The gums and conjunctiva, or tissues surrounding the eye, are the best place to assess your cat's color. This is a difficult judgment call and requires some experience to be accurate. All three tissues should be pink. Shades of blue, gray, yellow, or white indicate a circulatory or metabolic problem and you should call your veterinarian as soon as possible.

Regression: Your cat should make steady progress back to his old self after an anesthetic, dental, or surgical procedure. Your veterinarian can give you an idea of how long this should take. Complications may have developed if your cat backslides or regresses in his recovery. This is particularly important during recovery from orthopedic surgeries.

Vomiting: The vomiting your cat experiences after anesthesia or surgery may be the side effect of the anesthetic itself. Other causes include car sickness, over-feeding or gluttony on the part of your famished friend, antibiotics or other drugs, a "bug," food intolerance or diet change, progression of a disease, or a complication of the surgical procedure. Vomiting as a result of the anesthetic or car sickness should not occur more than once or twice. This vomiting can be minimized by only feeding your cat a very small meal when he first returns home.

Chapter 13
Pregnancy and Delivery

Reproduction and the Healthy Cat

The onset of puberty and sexual behavior in cats begins at about 5 to 9 months of age, and questions related to the cat's sex life make up a large portion of the calls to most small animal hospitals. For this reason, a few of the basics are included here.

Most, but not all cats that are sexually mature, indicate this through some changes in their behavior. For young males, this is through territorial urine spraying, roaming, and aggressive behavior towards other males who impinge on his domain. These types of behavior begin to appear even before some of the physical characteristics related to sexual maturity develop. Tomcats often develop prominent cheeks or *jowls*, and a broad head. Unaltered males are more muscular and may develop a greasy patch of fur at the base of their tail in a condition called *stud tail*.

Female cats are called *queens*, a name of which I have always approved, especially in consideration of my own two females. Queens reach sexual maturity at about the same age as males and females can become pregnant at the time of their first breeding, a fact that has been the consternation of many cat owners caught by surprise. Unlike dogs, there are no external physical signs of *estrus* in female cats: no bloody vaginal discharge and no swelling of the vulva. Female cats indicate that they are ready to be bred entirely through behavior designed to attract and encourage males.

A female cat beginning her estrous or *heat cycle* becomes restless and vocal. She rubs her head affectionately against her owner or any upright object, marking the owner and these objects with the oily secretions from the glands positioned on the relatively hairless areas below her ears on her forehead. A sexually receptive queen will roll on the floor or *tread* with her hind feet if you scratch the base of her tail. When treading, she alternately lifts her left and right rear feet in quick succession while raising her hind quarters in the air and crouching on her front legs. She might yowl a long and mournful guttural cry and wander around the house or sit at the door. Many people are unfamiliar with these normal estrous behaviors, and think their cat is ill or in pain.

At first, the period of sexual receptivity is very short and the time between these episodes is longer. If there is no successful mating, the hormones that induce this behavior will wane and for several days she will no longer seek out a male or act interested in mating. Eventually, the period of receptivity will last longer and she will go out of heat for only one or two days, only to quickly return to her estrous behaviors of crying, rolling, and treading.

Unlike dogs that exhibit signs of estrus only one, two, or perhaps three times a year, cats will continue in this pattern during most of the year. Cats will have more frequent estrous periods during January and the winter months, tapering off into the summer. The pattern of estrous cycles is influenced by the length of natural sunlight exposure, the breed of cat, and, of course, individual variation.

Not all female cats will exhibit the prominent behavior associated with sexual receptivity, very young females in particular. Owners of these cats are likely to let the cat out the back door as usual one morning and receive a surprise two months later. If kit-tens are not in your future, keep all female cats indoors and away from their male siblings, too, until they have been spayed.

Mating

Sexual intercourse itself is brief. The female will crouch and present her hindquarters to the male, who mounts her and grasps the loose skin on her neck with his teeth. Intromission and ejaculation occur, lasting only a few seconds. The female will emit a scream and turn on the male, hissing and spitting. She will then characteristically roll and lick her vulva for several minutes. This act will be repeated several more times over a few hours. After successfully mating, the female's ovaries will release eggs which will be fertilized by the male's sperm as they are encountered in her reproductive tract. Once pregnant, the cycle of estrous behavior stops.

Pregnancy and Delivery

The normal gestation time for cats is 64 to 69 days, roughly two months. Around the time for delivery or *queening*, the female will seek out a secluded nest. It may be the back of your closet, under the lilacs, in the hayloft, or in the center of your bed. There will usually be little fuss or bother, but a few

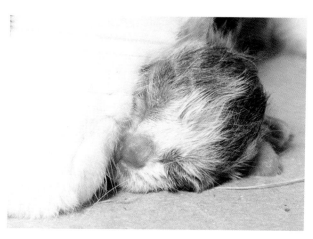

Two hours after birth.

covering their bodies. She will chew the *umbilical cord* to separate the placenta and unless you are there to intervene, she will more than likely eat it. Consuming the placenta doesn't seem to be a problem, unpleasant as that sounds.

Most mother cats stay with the kittens except for very short periods of time to eat and eliminate. (However, female cats can and do go into heat and can become pregnant again as little as 48 hours after delivering a litter.) Mothers will move the litter to a more secluded nest if the kittens are handled too often.

Mother cats rarely require assistance in the delivery of their kittens. Your most significant contribution to the birth will be to provide appropriate prenatal care to the mother. This should include the immunizations discussed earlier in the book (see page 15), and attention to her nutrition.

Pregnant cats should be fed a high-quality diet formulated specifically for kittens, beginning in the last third of the pregnancy when the fetuses are in their rapid growth stage. Continue to feed the mother this food until the kittens are weaned. The nutritional requirements for energy and protein for pregnant and nursing cats are about double those of a healthy nonpregnant female cat. You can meet these requirements by feeding your pregnant cat this diet. A diet formulated to support nonpregnant adult cats may be

pregnant queens will stay close to the owner. Cats can delay the onset of labor or halt the delivery process if the nest is disturbed. Just prior to delivery, her body temperature will drop to under 100°F (37.8°C).

Kittens are usually delivered after a few strong contractions that look like waves across her abdomen, with the whole litter being born in just a few hours. Some cats deliver part of the litter and then go out of labor for up to 24 hours before delivering the remaining kittens. This could be because of a lack of privacy during delivery, or because the kittens were conceived at different matings. Pauses in the delivery process are perfectly fine, but if your queen is in active labor and straining for more than 45 minutes without producing a kitten, you should call your veterinarian.

A placenta is usually passed immediately after each kitten is born. The female will lick each newborn to clean off the translucent membranes

Table 4

Signs of potential problems related to birth.

Problem	Possible causes
Bloody vaginal discharge	Before 8 weeks gestation: possible abortion or resorption of the litter.
	After 8 weeks gestation: premature delivery
Smelly vaginal discharge	Infected uterus; dead kitten.
Prolonged gestation	Dead fetus; earlier resorption; failure to conceive; inaccurate mating dates.
Straining to deliver more than 45 minutes	Uterus weak, tired; kitten too large to pass through birth canal; abortion.
Kitten stuck in birth canal	Too large to be delivered; kitten dead; uterus weak; mother fatigued.
Failure to pass placenta	Passed but mother consumed; retained placenta.
Hole in kitten's abdomen	Umbilical cord cut too close; hernia; congenital defect.
Deformed kitten	Congenital defect; genetic defect; infection *in utero*

inadequate in energy, protein, and minerals for the pregnant or nursing queen.

Although problems related to queening, or the delivery of kittens are rare, there are a few precautions that you should take. If you know the breeding dates for the mother, calculate the approximate delivery date on your calendar. Watch for any subtle signs of nesting behavior as this date approaches. You can check her body temperature, but this intrusion may delay the onset. Once labor has started, some owners call their veterinarian's office and let the staff know that the kittens are arriving, just in case of a problem.

Have some soft hand towels ready to help the mother remove the fetal membranes and dry off the kittens. If you need to tie off a kitten's umbilical cord, use thread or dental floss and a pair of scissors. Under no circumstances should you intervene in the delivery unless a problem arises. The mother will clean the kitten and detach the umbilical cord from the placenta in plenty of time, unless two kittens are born in quick succession. In this case, you can wipe the kittens' noses and mouths free from fluid and membranes, watch for breathing, and let her do her thing.

Problems with Delivery: Dystocia

Be aware of the few sign that could indicate a potential problem with the births. They are listed in Table 1. If you see any of these signs, you should consult your veterinarian.

Kittens are born covered by a set of thin, transparent membranes. Before birth, the kittens were suspended in a fluid enclosed by these membranes inside the uterus. A beltlike mass of blood vessels encircled the kitten's abdomen. This is the placenta. As a kitten passes through the birth canal, these membranes break and partially slide off, somewhat like the way you slide out of your socks. The mother licks the remnants of the membranes from around the kitten's face and body. The action of her tongue helps stimulate the kitten to breathe. What you will see are some initial gasps through the tiny mouth. Within seconds, the kitten will begin shallow, rapid respirations.

As the mother licks the kitten's body and encounters the umbilical cord, she chews it and frees the kitten from the placenta, the pulplike mass included with the fetal membranes. Soon after birth, check each kitten's umbilicus to make sure that the mother has not severed the attachment too closely, creating a hole in the abdomen. If this should happen, don't panic. Contact your veterinarian right away. Despite the high risk of infection or chance that a loop of intestine may drop through the hole, the kitten may do very well if the defect is closed surgically as soon as possible.

Sometimes the kittens come in such quick succession that the mother won't have time to attend to both. Two possible problems can occur. First, the membranes may not be cleared away from around the mouth and nose and the air passages may stay blocked. As the mother is busy alternating licking and cleaning each kitten, one may not receive enough stimulation to make it breathe on its own. This is a life-threatening problem. The second problem related to rapid births could be a failure of the mother to detach the placenta. This is not a life-threatening problem.

Attend to the first problem, the kitten's breathing. Gently wipe the kitten's face with your finger wrapped in a soft towel. In most cases, simply handling the kitten will stimulate it to breath. Wipe the kitten dry very carefully. It's very easy to tear a newborn's skin, especially around the flank folds and inner thighs. If the kitten doesn't start breathing, cradle her in a towel in the palms of your hands. Put her on her back with the hind feet toward you and gently swing the kitten downward toward the floor. This causes the fluid in the airways to flow upward and out the nose and mouth. Be especially careful not to fling the kitten out of your hands. I have seen overexcited owners assisting in Caesarean deliveries fling newborn puppies and kittens onto the floor by holding them improperly and swinging them too aggressively.

If you are confident that a kitten is breathing but its attachment to the placenta is still intact, tie the umbilical cord off tightly with a piece of dental floss or thread. Place one knot about an inch from the kitten's abdomen and a second one just a little bit beyond. Sever the cord between the two. Do not tie the cord if it is thick or irregular in diameter. A loop of intestine may have herniated through the abdominal wall and still be inside the umbilical cord. If you're not sure, call your veterinarian rather than make a serious misjudgment.

Neonatal Care

Even *primiparous* or *first-time* mothers instinctively know how to take care of the litter. Mothers don't leave their kittens except to eat or use the litterbox. Newborn kittens sleep continuously except to nurse. The mother stimulates them to urinate and defecate by licking, and she consumes the feces and urine.

Your role is to make sure that all the kittens are given attention and are nursing. The mother may push weak or sick kittens out of the nest. An inexperienced mother might abandon a kitten or the whole litter. Newborn kittens can't maintain their body temperature on their own and stay warm by snuggling against the mother and each other.

Abandoned kittens lose body heat very quickly. Once the body temperature drops below 96°F (35.6°C), the kitten can't absorb nutrients from its mother's milk or milk replacement formulas. These kittens can die within a few hours. Contact your veterinarian if any of your kittens are weak and/or nursing poorly. She will give you instructions on supplemental feeding and care. See page 44 for a description of how to make an incubator for orphaned or weak kittens and page 64 to review techniques for assisted-feeding.

Newborn kittens cry for one of three main reasons: They're cold, hungry, or constipated. The cold or hungry causes are easily to recognize and correct. If the kitten stops crying after nursing or being bottle-fed, then it was hungry. If you check its temperature and find it low, the crying will stop once the kitten is warm. But ceaseless crying in an otherwise warm and fed newborn kitten often means it's constipated. Contact your veterinarian for advice.

Newborn kittens spend most of their time sleeping, waking only briefly every hour or so to nurse. At about seventeen days of age, their ears and then their eyes will open and they will begin to explore the nest in a bobbing, uncoordinated, and very vocal fashion. By three weeks of age, the kittens' movements have gained coordination and they begin the play-behavior that is important in developing the fine motor skills necessary for hunting. The mother begins to wean the kittens at about five weeks, and at this time you should offer them a high-quality, very digestible canned kitten food.

Kittens should remain with their mother and littermates until eight or nine weeks of age.

Anatomy

It's really difficult to distinguish male kittens from female kittens until they are a couple of weeks old. Male kittens will have a round opening of the prepuce that is positioned directly under the anus. As a tom cat matures sexually, he will develop barbs or spines on his penis. Males usually have a larger head and prominent jowls if left unaltered. Females have a slit-like opening to the vulva under the anus, and will not develop jowls.

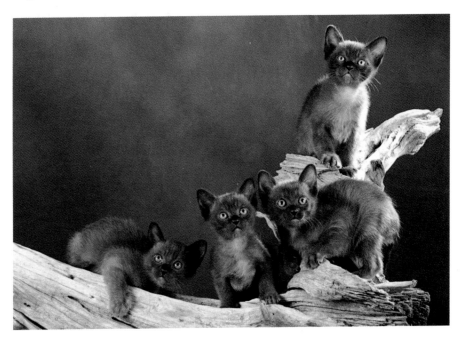

Chapter 14
Euthanasia

Euthanasia is also called "putting an animal to sleep." It is a nearly painless process. Most veterinarians give an injection of a powerful barbiturate anesthetic that first causes the animal to become unconscious, usually within about three seconds of injection.

Most of the time, this injection is given in a vein in the front leg. In very old cats or those with severe kidney or heart failure, the veins may be too fragile or collapsed because of low blood pressure. These cats can be given an injection directly into the heart. Your veterinarian will probably give this cat a relaxing dose of a sedative or a gas anesthetic first, to eliminate any possibility of anxiety or discomfort.

The drug acts on the brain and heart to cause the breathing and heartbeat to stop. There is no pain, except for the initial prick of the needle. That can be avoided too, if an intravenous catheter is already in place. Sometimes the animal may sigh, move, or void. These are just reflexes. The animal doesn't feel pain—or anything whatsoever. Death follows unconsciousness within two minutes.

Euthanasia is a difficult subject for everyone. As a veterinarian, I don't recommend putting a patient to sleep, except when I am absolutely certain that an animal is suffering, with little chance of recovery. The situation is rarely that black and white. Many of my clients will still ask me, "What would you do if this was your cat?" The decision depends on the cat's illness and quality of life, but also the relationship between the owner and the pet, the relationship with the family, a person's philosophy related to pets and the human-animal bond, the animal's age, and unfortunately, economics. I can only advise you. I don't want you to regret your decision, thinking afterwards that it was too soon, or delayed too long.

Grieving will be a natural and necessary part of accepting the loss of a pet. Many support groups have been organized within communities, veterinary schools, and local mental health organizations to help people go through what can be a very painful process. Your veterinarian may know of a support group or an individual who provides counseling.

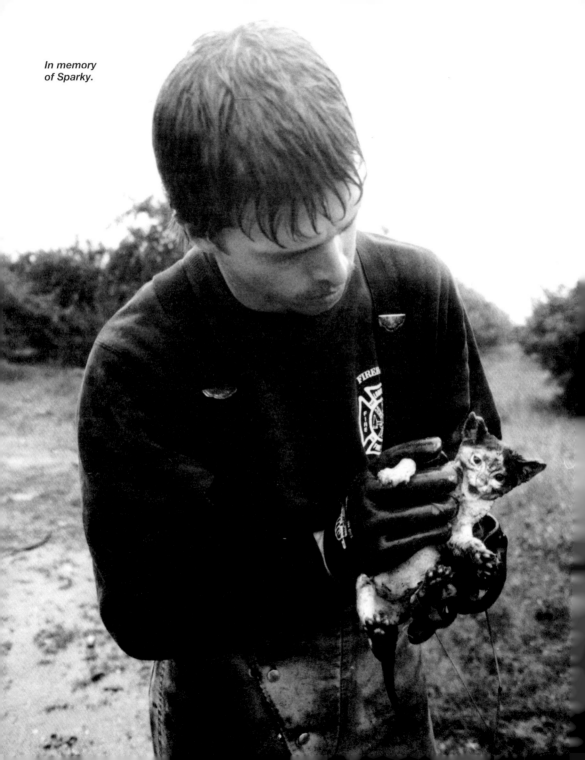

*In memory
of Sparky.*

Chapter 15

Maladies From A to Z

This section is not meant to be a manual for diagnosis and home treatment for your cat, but rather a detailed written explanation of the diseases, procedures, and nursing care that your veterinarian has probably already explained to you. Whether you are participating in a long convalescence at home or simply need to have this information available to mull over at a later time, this book should serve either purpose.

The discussion of cat diseases is done in an encyclopedic manner. The information is similar to what I might tell a cat owner about a disease, diagnosis, and prognosis for each condition. In that manner. Thus it is somewhat biased towards my personal medical opinion and clinical experience. You may wish to ask your veterinarian about a difference in what he or she tells you and what is written here if you are concerned.

This is not intended to be a complete treatise on feline medicine. The diseases discussed here are the "big hitters" for cats, and I have included a few that have more significance to humans and one or two of interest because of their oddity.

A

Abcess

An abscess is an accumulation of pus contained in a pocket under the skin. It's often the result of a puncture wound to the skin, and in cats is almost always a consequence of a bite from another cat. Cat abscesses are common on the forelegs, head, neck, and at the base of the tail, not surprisingly all common target sites for other cats to bite! Ragged-eared tomcats wear battle scars on their front legs, head, and neck as testimony to their territorial behavior.

Bite wounds are not the only cause for abscesses. Any puncture to the skin introduces bacteria from the soil and the environment into the tissues below. In the western United States, foxtails or plant awns from wild oats pierce the skin and migrate through tissues causing draining tracts and abscesses.

Once the skin is punctured, a natural barrier to infection is lost. Bacteria from the mouth or environment and fragments of hair, dirt, and debris are introduced into the deeper tissues. The puncture wound seals over quickly and the skin heals even as the bacteria begin to multiply and cause an infection. This infection results in a massive influx of pus cells into the area to gobble up the bacteria. The immune system usually walls off the area to prevent the infection from spreading under the skin. In this manner, the pus and bacteria are contained within a pocket. Sometimes you can feel a soft, fluctuant pocket under the skin. If you part the fur, you might see the

Foxtails can pierce the skin.

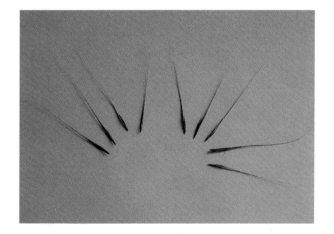

tiny puncture wounds or might feel a scab.

Abscesses are very painful. The overlying skin becomes stretched from the pressure of the expanding pocket. Bacterial toxins and products of inflammation are released that cause pain, swelling, redness and heat. Abscesses on limbs can be so painful that your cat won't bear any weight on the leg and many owners think the leg is broken. Abscesses are accompanied by high fever and lack of appetite.

Antibiotics alone are not effective in treating an infection that has progressed to the abscess stage. The hallmark of treatment for abscesses is *drainage*. This can be accomplished by surgically placing drains such as Penrose or umbilical-tape drains (see page 82). If the skin over the abscess is extensively damaged, it may need to be removed in a surgical procedure called *debridement*. If the abscess has ruptured through a large opening and drainage can be maintained by compressing, placement of a drain may not be necessary. If the overlying skin heals too quickly, the abscess reforms.

Once drainage is established, treatment continues with hot compressing two or three times a day. You may also need to flush the wound with an appropriate antiseptic solution. Oral antibiotics are given for 7 to 14 days. Your cat should be force fed if will not eat on its own.

A recurrence of an abscess in the same location may be due to inadequate drainage, spreading of the infection along deep tissue planes, improper or ineffective antibiotic dosing, or bacterial resistance. Do not underestimate the possibility that your cat may have been bitten in the same place again! This is very common. The consequences of abscesses include the spreading of the infection to other tissues or organs such as the kidney and urinary tract, liver, joints, heart, or lungs. Because cat bites are almost always the cause of abscesses, cats with abscesses are at risk for contracting serious cat viruses such as feline leukemia virus and feline immunodeficiency virus.

Acne

Just like teenagers, cats are plagued by acne. The chin blemishes appear exactly as you would expect—they are raised, white pimples that rupture easily, leaving a crater that sometimes bleeds. These defects can be tracts or fistulas that extend deeply into the tissues. In milder cases, there are only blackheads.

No one knows why some cats develop feline acne. One postulate is that the chin becomes irritated and dirty from eating out of a bowl with steeply sloped sides. If a cat is prone to developing feline acne, feed this cat on a flat plate. The fur should be clipped away so that the chin can be cleaned gently with an antiseptic and treated with a drying agent. Oral or topical antibiotics are given. This condition tends to recur.

Anterior Uveitis

Inflammation of the forward portion of the eye is called anterior uveitis. It can be caused by trauma or a blow to the eye when a cat is hit by a car; bacterial, fungal or viral infections; cancer, toxins, or autoimmune disease. The cornea or clear front part of the eye; the fluid between the cornea and the iris; the colored iris, and lens, or all three parts may be affected. It may be difficult to assess the iris or lens because of edema or water accumulation in the cornea, causing it to appear an opaque light blue, or the presence of blood or pus that block our ability to examine deeper into the eye.

The treatment and prognosis depends upon the cause. If the anterior uveitis is caused by a systemic disease, diagnosis and treatment of the primary disease is paramount. Anterior uveitis alone is treated by a combination of topical medications to control inflammation, infection, pain, a secondary glaucoma, adhesions or dislocation of the lens, or spread of the inflammatory process to involve deeper eye structures. Topical medication may include an injection into the sclera or white portion of the eye that allows for a constant slow release of the drug over a longer period of time. Oral antibiotics and anti-inflammatories may be used.

Asthma

Asthma is a respiratory disease that, like its counterpart in humans, is probably an allergic or hypersensitivity response to an environmental substance. This includes pollens, molds, house dust, aerosol sprays, litterbox dust, or deodorants, cigarette smoke or flea products. The list is exhaustive and rarely can the inciting cause(s) be identified with certainty. Several of my asthmatic feline patients would get worse during the winter holidays when the Christmas tree came indoors. One patient went into an acute crisis after the owner inadvertently used a sprinkle-on carpet deodorizer.

The hallmark clinical sign of asthma is cough. It is not the only cause. A complete work-up is necessary to determine the cause of any cough. This includes blood tests: a complete blood count and heartworm test, fecal examination for lung parasites and radiographs. It may be necessary to do an endoscopy or a bronchial wash to obtain a sample of the fluid and cells that line the respiratory passages before a definitive diagnosis can be made.

Asthma is treated with corticosteriods to control the allergic response and antibiotics if the doctor suspects a secondary infection. An attempt should be made to eliminate any potentially inciting causes—for instance, don't allow your cat in the room if you use hairspray. Switch to a minimally dusty cat litter. Quit smoking.

Asthma is a potentially fatal disease. While the cough and changes seen on radiographs can be controlled nicely with medication in most cats, relapses can and do occur. They can range anywhere from an increase in the frequency or severity of coughing to acute respiratory distress and asphyxiation. Asthmatic cats should be rechecked at least once a year.

C

Calicivirus

This is a respiratory virus found in almost all cats and kittens. It is one of several viruses included in routine kittenhood and adult

An autoclave uses steam heat and pressure to sterilize instruments.

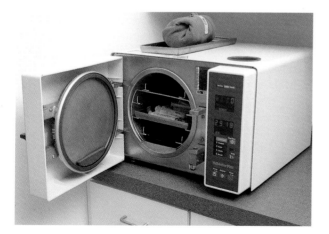

vaccination programs. It causes the upper respiratory disease signs of sneezing and watery nasal discharge. Calicivirus infections often cause ulcerations in the mouth on the hard palate and tongue. These are painful and afflicted cats don't eat because of the pain and inability to smell their food. There may be a fever. In rare cases, a secondary pneumonia may develop. Once the virus has infected the tissues of the respiratory tract, normally harmless bacteria that live on these tissues begin to proliferate and cause disease. The watery discharge becomes thicker and opaque. Conjunctivitis may be a secondary problem.

Antiviral medications are not practical. Treatment involves supportive care: antibiotics both orally and in the eyes, fluids, force feeding, quiet, and rest. Calicivirus infection is not usually fatal except in very young kittens that become very dehydrated and are anorectic for several days.

Vaccination is highly effective in controlling the disease. Although it is not 100 percent effective in prevention, the disease is not as severe in cats that have been properly vaccinated. Kittens and cats that have been vaccinated can still get the disease if they are exposed to a large dose of the virus under such circumstances as when boarding and stressed. Once over an initial infection, most cats become chronic carriers who can pass the virus on to kittens or who can have an occasional mild recrudescence of the disease.

Cancer

Any cell or tissue in the body can become cancerous, it doesn't matter what species of animal it's in. Cells growing in a dish in the laboratory can transform into cancer cells. In cats, the most common locations for tumors are the gastrointestinal tract (adenocarcinoma), the skin (squamous cell carcinomas, mast cell and basal cell tumors) and associated structures, (mammary tumors) and the immune system (lymphoma and leukemia).

Cells become cancerous when they lose all regulation over how they divide and organize into tissues, what function they perform, and what substances they secrete. Cancers can be malignant—that is, spread to other locations—or be benign. Benign tumors stay in one place. They cause harm by disrupting the architecture and function of the adjacent normal structures.

Just as in people, cancer in animals can grow slowly and have little effect until the disease is widespread or deeply invasive. There may be little physical or laboratory evidence to suggest cancer. They can also grow rapidly, making what seemed to be a healthy cat very sick, very quickly.

When a diagnosis of cancer is made, it is important to know all the organs that have been affected.

Blood and urine analysis, radiographs, ultrasonography, biopsy, and bone marrow evaluation are used to "stage" the disease. Staging the cancer helps the doctor decide whether or not to recommend treatment, and gives an idea of the probable outcome of treatment. *Cancer is not always fatal.*

In small animals, cancer is treated using surgery, anticancer drugs, radiation, hyperthermia, immune therapy, and combinations of all of them. Some cancers respond better than others to the same form of treatment, so it's important to know exactly what the cancer is in order to make the right choice on what to use.

A lot of drugs used against human cancers are also used in animals. We don't see the same degree of side effects because veterinarians use lower doses and fewer numbers of drugs at the same time. Cost is a big issue in cancer treatment for pets, as is the quality of life of the patient. A less aggressive program seems appropriate, because the goal is to maintain the best possible quality of life and companionship with the owner until the end. The decision to treat many serious and extensive cancers is sometimes made in order to give the owner the necessary time to accept the death of their cat.

New and promising anticancer treatments are used in veterinary medicine every year. Many teaching hospitals participate in drug-company-sponsored research programs studying the effectiveness of new protocols on animal cancers. Drugs are often supplied at no cost to the client, and the cat lives comfortably secure at home with the owner while participating in such studies. This is one way owners can receive financial and advanced medical assistance for their cats with cancer.

Cardiomyopathy (congestive heart failure)

By breaking this word down into its parts: *cardio-*, meaning heart, *-myo-*, meaning muscle, and *-pathy,* meaning disorder, you know that this is a disease of the heart muscle. A form of cardiomyopathy also occurs in other species, including dogs and people. In cats, the two most important types of cardiomyopathy recognized by veterinary cardiologists are classified by the physical changes that have occurred in the heart muscle. *Dilated cardiomyopathy* is the most severe form and is most often associated with a deficiency in the dietary amino acid *taurine*. It used to be a more common problem in cats until pet food companies began adding a lot more *taurine* to their foods. *Hypertrophic cardiomyopathy* is the other most common form. (There are others with subtle differences which are unimportant here.) The cause is unknown. Hypertrophic cardiomyopathy is a common complication in hyperthyroid cats, but there are plenty of affected cats with no other apparent associations.

Cats with cardiomyopathy may not have any clinical signs, even in severe cases, if the disease has progressed slowly and the cat's body has had time to adapt to the diminished "cardiac reserve." Clinical signs that are usually seen are weakness, depression, inappetence, difficulty breathing, cough, and collapse. Within the circulatory system of a cat with cardiomyopathy, the anatomic and physiologic conditions are ripe for the formation of large blood clots, a condition called thromboembolism. These blood clots can form and lodge anywhere in the circulatory system, most notably at the final branching of the large vessel that supplies blood to the rear limbs. If thromboembolism does occur, there may be severe pain in the hind legs. But be aware that even if there are no outward signs, cardiomyopathy can cause sudden death.

The diagnosis is based on a history or report of problems by the owner, physical examination, radiographs, and an ultrasound evaluation of the heart. Sometimes angiography will be needed. Blood tests are necessary to determine how severely other organs have been affected by the heart disease, to identify a cause if possible, and to aid in therapy.

A measurement of the blood-taurine level is important in cases of dilated cardiomyopathy. Not every cat that is diagnosed with dilated cardiomyopathy will have a taurine level below what is considered to be normal. While cats eating cheap, improperly cooked commercial cat foods, home-cooked diets, vegetarian diets, and exclusively organ-meat diets are at greatest risk, many cats with dilated cardiomyopathy are not eating a diet deficient in taurine because commercial pet foods are supplemented. These cats may have different requirements for taurine, or may process this amino acid differently from other cats. Taurine deficiency by itself is probably not the sole cause of this form of cardiomyopathy. Veterinary scientists are still working to determine the other factors involved.

Treatment depends upon the type of cardiomyopathy. Medications control the heart rate and blood pressure, improve the heart's ability to pump blood, and control other complications to organs caused by the heart disease. Cats with the dilated form of cardiomyopathy are given oral supplements of taurine, regardless of the blood taurine level. Treatment may also include a salt-restricted diet. Hyperthyroidism will be corrected if that is the initiating cause.

In most instances, cardiomyopathy is a very severe problem and the prognosis is guarded. Fortunately, many cats who in past years would have died from

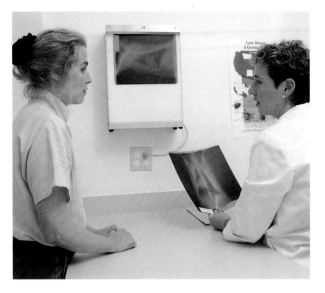

Conjunctivitis

This is an inflammation of the delicate tissues lining the inside of the eyelids. Bacteria, viruses, irritants, chemicals, and trauma initiate the inflammation. Conjunctivitis can occur alone or in association with upper respiratory infections. Signs of conjunctivitis include blinking, redness, and swelling along the eyelids, and watery to cloudy, thick discharge. Conjunctivitis sometimes seems to itch because the animal will rub its eyes. Topicals with or without oral antibiotics are used for treatment. Depending upon the cause, conjunctivitis can be difficult to cure.

Take the time to learn as much as you need to in order to understand your cat's diagnostic tests, diagnosis, treatments, and prognosis. This may mean scheduling a specific appointment with the doctor so that you may discuss the case uninterrupted.

dilated cardiomyopathy, now survive and can be taken off medication and taurine supplements. Cats with cardiomyopathy require frequent reevaluation and monitoring of their heart medication. See also *Hyperthyroidism, Thromboembolism.*

Chlamydia

This very primitive bacteria causes conjunctivitis in kittens and cats. Topical antibiotics in the eye are used for treatment, but chlamydial conjunctivitis is very difficult to cure. Classic chlamydial infections recur over and over again after ill-defined periods of quiescence. Antibiotics given orally for a long period of time sometimes help to lengthen those periods of "remission." Chlamydial conjunctivitis is transmissible to people; wash your hands after treating your cat. See also *Conjunctivitis.*

Constipation (obstipation, fecal impaction, megacolon)

Just like any other animal, cats experience constipation. This can result from inadequate amounts of dietary fiber in the diet, inadequate water intake, or excessive hair in the stool. Obstruction of the rectum by a fractured and collapsed pelvis or tumor will prevent effective elimination. Limb and spinal fractures, or simply pain, will inhibit a cat from getting into the litterbox or assuming the necessary position for defecation. (Dirty litterboxes or competition for the litterbox in multiple cat households will do the same.) Secondarily, severe constipation called obstipation occurs with severe illness and dehydration. Some drugs, particularly diuretics (drugs that induce water loss in the urine), promote constipation.

In its most severe form, a disease in geriatric cats called megacolon or fecal impaction is the result of the loss of nerve function to the colon and rectum. Normal contractions of varying magnitude move feces through the colon and rectum. If these do not occur, the feces remains in the rectum. These cats have lost most of the ability to sense fullness and the need to defecate. They continue to eat and produce fecal material that impacts the entire length of the large bowel. If the innervation isn't completely lost, the cat strains as the stretching of the colon and rectum becomes uncomfortable. They do not eliminate at all, or they pass only small amounts of feces. Some of these cats actually develop diarrhea. The watery stool leaks around the fecal mass obstructing the colon. Overstretching the walls of the large bowel further damages their ability to contract. That's why this condition is sometimes called *mega*colon. It's a big deal. . .

As feces sit in the colon, water is reabsorbed back into the body making the feces drier and passage more difficult. Severely constipated cats are dehydrated and depressed. A combination of multiple enemas and manual removal of the impacted feces is necessary. Manual removal requires general anesthesia for the comfort and cooperation of the cat.

Treatment for simple constipation includes petrolatum-based flavored laxatives, supplemental fiber laxatives, and high fiber diets and grooming. Petrolatum laxatives work by lubricating the feces to assist in their passage. Fiber laxatives and fiber diets work by increasing the bulk of the stool by imbibing water into the fecal mass. The increase in fecal bulk stimulates contractions and elimination occurs. Naturally, some normal nerve function must be present for these to work at all. Both veterinary preparations of fiber capsules and human fiber laxatives are used for supplements. These are not as effective as feeding a high fiber diet on a daily basis. Fiber supplements change the flavor and texture of the food so that some cats won't eat them. There is also a tendency to forget to add the supplement every day. Prescription-type fiber diets provide a more consistent level of fiber and much better palatability. And the owner doesn't have to remember to add extra fiber.

Initially, cats with megacolon are given petrolatum-based laxatives and are fed a fiber supplement or high-fiber diet. This will work as long as there is some residual nerve function in the large bowel. When that goes and the cat doesn't, a highly digestible, low-fiber diet is fed so that as little fecal material as possible is produced. The owner is taught to give enemas regularly at home.

A surgical procedure to remove the diseased portion of the large bowel can be performed, but this procedure is not without risk.

Chronic diarrhea and incontinence are complications. In the hands of a skilled surgeon, some cats have benefitted greatly from this surgery.

Corneal Ulcer

A defect or crater in the outer layers of the cornea is called an ulcer. Ulcers are irregular in shape and depth. The edges of the ulcer tend to lift and peel away, creating a larger defect. Corneal ulcers are often the result of an abrasion or rubbing on the cornea due to trauma, such as being hit by a car or having a foreign body like a foxtail or plant awn embedded in the conjunctiva rub on the surface of the eye. Some ulcers can be seen just by looking at the cornea. Most of the time, a drop of dye called fluorescein is instilled and the eye is examined using a black light. A corneal ulcer will glow apple green.

Treatment involves removing the diseased tissue so that new corneal cells can grow over the defect. Antibiotics are given topically and orally and medication is used to control pain. If the corneal ulcer is very deep, the cornea may rupture. To protect the eye from rupturing from a deep ulceration, the eyelids can be temporarily sutured closed with one or two stitches and medications carefully instilled behind the closure. Alternatively, the third eyelid or nictitating membrane may be drawn up over the cornea and sutured in place to act as a bandage over the ulcer. Thirdly, the entire ulcer may need to be removed sur-gically and the defect closed with tiny sutures.

Most corneal ulcers heal quickly and uneventfully. Severe ulcers can result in an infection spreading to the deeper tissues of the eye. It is important to give medications faithfully and to recheck the ulcer frequently until healed.

Cuterebra Larvae

These parasites in the skin are the larvae or maggot of the fly *cuterebra*. The fly lays its sticky eggs on the long blades of grass around burrows in the ground. Small animals such as rabbits passing through the opening to the burrow or cats who stick their heads into the burrows looking for the rabbits, get the eggs caught on their fur around their head and face. The eggs hatch and the larvae crawls down into the fur and burrow into the skin. It creates a cyst that grows larger as the larva enlarges to almost an inch (2.3 cm) in length. The parasite breathes through an opening in the skin. Eventually the cyst ruptures and the larva drops out to complete its life cycle.

By themselves, the larva and the cyst don't cause much of a problem to the cat except for a mild localized infection. However, most cat owners understandably object when they see a huge maggot moving under the skin and request its removal. This should be done only by a veterinarian because rupture of the maggot can cause an anaphylactic reaction.

D

Dermatophytosis: See *Ringworm*

Diabetes Mellitus (DM)

Distinct from its function in digestion, the pancreas secretes several other hormones, including one called insulin. Insulin is the hormone that drives glucose, a kind of sugar, into cells. Glucose is the major fuel source for all tissues. Without insulin, tissues starve until alternative fuels are manufactured from fat stores.

Diabetes mellitus is a disease in which the body doesn't have adequate amounts of insulin. This is called Type I or insulin-dependent diabetes. There is a second kind of diabetes called Type II or noninsulin dependent diabetes where the body actually has plenty of insulin but it doesn't work properly. Diabetes mellitus is a very important endocrine disease in cats.

Type I DM is the classically recognized disease. Type I diabetic cats are usually very thin, or on their way to being thin because of significant weight loss. They drink a lot of water and subsequently urinate large volumes. They may have enormous appetites. One diabetic patient of mine stole a whole chicken off a neighbor's barbecue grill. As the disease progresses, diabetic cats become weak and may vomit. Dehydration, ketosis, and coma precede death.

In Type II or noninsulin dependent diabetes there is plenty of insulin being secreted by the pancreas, but the insulin is not effective in driving sugar into cells. Type II diabetic cats are often but not always, obese. They may drink a lot of water and urinate frequently, but they do not have ketosis.

After a meal, the amount of glucose in the blood will go up. In a normal animal, insulin will drive the glucose into the tissues, maintaining the amount of sugar in the blood within a narrow range. In diabetic patients, because the insulin isn't available or doesn't work properly, blood sugars stay very high. There's so much sugar in the blood that it is excreted by the kidneys in the urine. The sugar in the urine is a very good fuel for bacteria too, so many diabetic cats have urinary tract infections.

Both types of diabetes occur in middle-aged to older cats. Diabetes is suggested by the history and physical examination of the cat and confirmed after measuring high levels of glucose in the blood and urine on repeated tests. A full blood analysis, including complete blood count and chemistry panel, are done to see if there is other organ dysfunction. If the urinalysis suggests infection, the urine is cultured for bacteria.

If the cat is very sick, the initial treatment to stabilize the blood sugar and correct dehydration and ketosis is done in the hospital. These conditions can be very difficult to correct, and many of these cats are also in some degree of kidney failure. Their condition will initially be very unstable.

Most diabetic cats are not seriously ketotic and unstable. There are two courses of treatment possible, depending upon which type of diabetes the veterinarian feels is most likely the problem. The type of diabetes can be confirmed by doing a special type of test where the patient is given a large intravenous dose of glucose or the hormone glucagon and the blood insulin levels are measured several times. Naturally, if the cat is a Type I diabetic, no insulin will be produced in response to either stimulus.

Most veterinarians don't routinely use these response tests to type the diabetes. If the cat is stable and the need for insulin injections is in question, the veterinarian may manage the diabetes by manipulating the diet to see if the blood sugar will stabilize and the diabetes resolves if the cat loses weight. Insulin injections are unnecessary for Type II DM because there is plenty of insulin. If one of the reasons for the insulin not working in Type II diabetics is tied in with being overweight, these cats go on a diet! Diabetes management using controlled amounts of fiber in the diet is often enough to control blood sugar levels all by itself. Sometimes oral medications that lower blood sugar are used in conjunction with fiber diets. Over time, the diabetes can resolve.

The only way to treat Type I DM is to give daily injections of insulin. This isn't very hard to do—see page 75 for a description of the technique. Usually a fixed dose is first prescribed and the owner gives the cat this dose once or twice a day for about a week. Then the cat comes back to the hospital and the blood sugar is measured several times a day to see if the dose is correct. We call serial measurements like this a *glucose curve*. Glucose curves are the benchmark for evaluating effectiveness of the insulin.

Adjustments in the type of insulin, dose, and dose schedule are made based on glucose curves. Some veterinarians will have owners obtain a small urine sample and check it for sugar every day or every few days. If the dose of insulin is appropriate, the blood sugars will stay low enough to prevent sugar from appearing in the urine. See page 51 for a method for catching a urine sample.

Dietary management plays a big role in the treatment of Type I DM also. Diabetic cats should be fed a prescription-type fiber diet. The addition of fiber to the diet makes it much easier to regulate blood sugars and helps the insulin that is given to be more efficient. Forget about variety—diabetic cats should be fed the same food every day. They should never be fed semi-moist diets because of the sugar content. Most importantly, diabetic cats should eat, so that there is sugar in the blood for the insulin to work on, otherwise the insulin injection can result in hypoglycemic seizures as the blood sugar drops precipitously.

There are many serious complications with Type I DM, beginning with the initial ketosis and dehydration that is present in a few cases. Once daily insulin treatment is begun, the most common complication is hypoglycemia or low blood sugar, either from insulin overdose or from the cat not eating after getting the insulin. Hypoglycemia is fairly easy to spot; the cat will be weak. Hypoglycemia can be reversed by rubbing Karo syrup on the gums. Then contact your veterinarian right away.

Having a diabetic cat can have a significant impact on the owner's life. The initial diagnosis and stabilization period may take several weeks and means several trips to the veterinary hospital. Insulin is not very expensive, but the lab tests and cost of veterinary care are substantial. Once stabilized, these costs drop dramatically.

Having a diabetic pet means the owner must be home every day at insulin time. Vacations and separations from the owner can mean that the diabetes becomes unregulated because of the stress and change in daily routine. Short-term unregulated diabetes doesn't have to be life-threatening, but it may take some effort to get things back on track, and ketosis is always a risk. This can be minimized by having a cat-sitter or a special boarding arrangement with a veterinarian.

Untreated diabetes is a slowly fatal disease, during which time the cat doesn't feel very well. Despite the costs and potential complications, managing a diabetic cat can be extremely rewarding for everyone. Once the diabetes is stabilized and the cat is feeling well, daily insulin injections are simple and routine, and the cat can have a full life.

Diaphragmatic Hernia

The diaphragm is a broad, flat, thin but tough muscle that separates the chest cavity from the abdominal cavity. It is attached to the body wall along its circumference, forming the partition. Aside from its function of dividing the body and thus organizing the internal organs, the diaphragm has an important role in respiration. During inspiration, the diaphragm moves backwards creating a relative vacuum inside the chest cavity that allows the lungs to expand with air. On the abdominal side of the diaphragm immediately lies the liver. Several major vessels pass through the diaphragm bringing oxygen-rich blood to tissues or oxygen-depleted blood back to the heart. Vessels carrying lymph fluid and large nerves also course the diaphragm.

If the diaphragm separates from the body wall anywhere along its attachment, a diaphragmatic hernia results. The body is no longer partitioned into chest and abdominal cavities; instead there is now a communication between these two spaces. Organs from the abdomen, usually portions of the liver and gastrointestinal tract, are displaced into the chest. This leaves less room for the lungs and heart. Expansion of the lungs during inspiration is further compromised by the incomplete and inefficient motion of the diaphragm. Displaced organs will obstruct the blood flow in the vessels that pass through the diaphragm and cause plasma to leak from the vessels into the now confluent chest and abdominal cavities. This causes added compression on the organs, especially the lungs and heart.

Diaphragmatic hernias are most often the result of traumatic injuries, such as automobile accidents and falls. On rare occasions, the diaphragm can rupture secondarily to severe thoracic or abdominal infections. Congenital malformation of the diaphragm can result in hernias from the time of birth.

The cardinal sign of diaphragmatic hernia is dyspnea, or labored breathing. Many cats with this condition go undiagnosed for a long time, especially if the rent in the diaphragm is small and the organs slip in and out. These cats may exhibit signs only with exertion or stress. Some diaphragmatic hernias are diagnosed when an animal undergoes surgery and experiences anesthetic complications.

Treatment for diaphragmatic hernias involves surgical reattachment. The displaced organs are returned to their proper position. If the blood supply to the displaced organs has been compromised and the tissue is severely damaged, it may need to be removed. Scarring of the displaced organs in their abnormal position and hemorrhage are two serious complications to this surgery. If damage to the diaphragm is extensive, repair may be impossible and synthetic grafting material is used to replace the muscle.

Anesthesia is very difficult for these patients who must be assisted to breathe during the procedure, either manually by an assistant or with a mechanical respirator. However, prognosis is surprisingly good, despite the risks and severity of the condition.

E

Ear Mites

These tiny insect parasites live in and around the ears and neck of dogs and cats. They are highly contagious from animal to animal. Feeding on skin scales and secretions, ear mites cause intense itching as they scurry around inside the ear canals. Kittens are most likely to be infected, catching mites from their mothers who often don't show any clinical signs.

After a period of time, the ear canals become packed with a black, waxy, granular debris that looks a lot like coffee grounds. There may be a secondary yeast or bacterial infection and severe dermatitis around the head and neck from the self-trauma associated with the itching and scratching.

The ears should be thoroughly flushed to remove the debris. Topical medications are instilled to control the secondary bacterial infection and kill the mites. A drug called ivermectin is given orally or subcutaneously in one or two doses to eradicate the infection. Although this drug is currently not approved for use with cats for this problem, it has been widely and safely used. Alternatively, topical medications must be given for one to four weeks. Because the mites live on the fur around the head and neck, flea-control products should be applied to kill them so they can't reinfect the ears.

It is very important that all cats and dogs in the household be treated for ear mites at the same time, whether or not they are showing signs, and whether or not mites are found on examination or on swabs of the debris. If not, the mites will persist in the household and contribute to chronic otitis problems. Ear mites do not infect people.

Eosinophilic Granuloma Complex (EGC, linear granuloma, rodent ulcer)

A bizarre skin disease, this complex has no known cause and a variety of presentations. The classic disease EGC can be divided into three types. The most alarming is one that involves the development of raised, red, leathery plaque lesions, commonly on the forelegs, chest, and sides. A second type is similar, but the lesions are smaller and can vary from the raised plaque form to simply a linear array of scabs limited in location to the back of the hind legs. The third form and probably the most common is called rodent ulcer, a name implying that the disease is caused by rodents like rats and mice, which it is not. In rodent ulcer, the margin of the upper lip between the gingiva and skin erodes away, creating a crater that can extend for some considerable distance along the lip.

EGC doesn't seem overtly painful, except for the rodent ulcer type which can keep cats from eating. It's probably pruritic or itchy, because cats groom and lick themselves excessively in these areas. They may then become infected by the normal garden-variety skin bacteria because of this self-trauma.

There have been a number of attempts to explain the cause of these lesions. Biopsies show an influx of the white blood cell called an eosinophil into the tissues. What prompts these cells to leave the circulation and enter tissues in such large numbers is unknown. Eosinophils are an important component in allergic responses. No one has demonstrated that allergies to foods, pollens, chemicals, fleas, or contact substances are involved. One popular yet unproven theory is that rodent ulcer is caused by an allergy to the dyes in plastic food bowls. Feline leukemia virus infection, our usual nemesis, has not been implicated either.

EGC is usually a problem for adult cats. The diagnosis is made based on physical examination and biopsy, if necessary. Treatment aims at eliminating any known causes of allergic or hypersensitivity response, especially flea infestation. Sometimes a trial for food allergy is recommended. The large plaques are treated by combining oral corticosteroids and injections of corticosteroids into the lesions themselves. Surgery and radiation therapy is also used. Although not a fatal disease, the prognosis is guarded because it's difficult to resolve large plaques and the condition tends to recur.

F

Feline Immunodeficiency Virus (FIV)

A relatively recent discovery, FIV is very similar to the human immunodeficiency virus. FIV is not transmissible to humans or any other animals. It appears to be transmitted between cats only by bite wounds, unlike FeLV, which can be transmitted through casual contact. The virus does not cross the placenta.

Unlike feline leukemia virus, scientists don't know much about what happens with the virus once it enters the body. We do know that cats infected with FIV can harbor the virus inside their bodies for several years before any disease consequences develop. Because the virus is difficult to transmit and because it can take many years for the cat to actually get sick, the significance of infection is not completely known.

Feline immunodeficiency virus is associated with diseases that one might expect with a suppressed immune system: chronic infections including respiratory and gastrointestinal, chronic and severe periodontal disease, chronic and recurrent skin infections, to name a few. It has also been implicated in some cancers and some neurologic diseases.

FIV-positive cats should be monitored closely for signs of illness, including yearly complete blood count and chemistry panels for organ dysfunction. There is no reason not to treat FIV-infected cats for chronic illnesses. Unless the cat is aggressive toward other cats, isolation is not necessary. There is no vaccine available at this time.

Feline Infectious Anemia

Sometimes called *Haemobartonellosis*, this disease is caused by *Haemobartonella*, a primitive bacteri-alike parasite that attaches to the surface of red blood cells. This attachment causes damage to the red cells, making them fragile so that they break apart, and stimulates the immune system, which attacks the altered red cells and removes them from circulation. These animals become very anemic.

Haemobartonella is transferred between cats by the exchange of blood during fights. The organism is probably widespread throughout the cat population and goes undetected unless a cat actually becomes sick. The parasite can be seen on blood smears made for a complete blood count, but it looks a lot like granules of stain or normal cat red-blood-cell structures, so it isn't recognized. Healthy cats can carry very small numbers of Haemobartonella organisms in their blood. For reasons not quite understood, the parasite begins to multiply and cause disease in some cats. Many of these cats are co-infected with FeLV and FIV.

Cats with feline infectious anemia appear weak, pale, and lack an appetite. There may be a fever. The diagnosis is made by observing the organism on blood smears, but this can be difficult because the number of Haemobartonella organisms can wax and wane. These cats should be tested for FIV and FeLV.

Haemobartonellosis can be treated with antibiotics, corticosteriods, and transfusions. There is some debate about whether cats are ever cured of the infection. Certainly some become chronic carriers that pass it on to others.

Haemobartonella is not transmissible to humans. Dogs can become infected with their own species of this parasite.

Feline Infectious Peritonitis

This virus is one of several in a group called Coronaviruses that most often cause nonfatal diarrhea in kittens and adult cats. FIP virus is different from others in this group because it infects the immune system cells called macrophages that are found scattered in all tissues of the body, especially the blood vessels that nourish the organs and walls of the chest and abdominal cavities. Antibodies are produced that attach to the virus. This stimulates the approach of white blood cells that eat up these complexes. The ensuing inflammation usually, but not always, causes a tremendous outpouring of fluid into the chest and abdomen.

Because macrophages are found everywhere, the virus also targets the liver, kidneys, eyes, brain, and spinal cord, causing more inflammation. It can also affect the uterus, causing abortions and weak kittens.

FIP virus is passed in the feces of cats that are infected but not sick. Cats inhale or consume the virus after using litterboxes or defecation spots also used by the virus-shedding cats. There may be a sexual transmission also.

The virus can survive in the environment for several weeks. No one knows why some cats get sick and some don't. Just like human influenza viruses, there is more than one strain of FIP virus. Some strains are stronger or more virulent than others and it is these strains that are probably responsible for the clinical disease. Many cats are also infected with FeLV and FIV which suppress their immune system and make them more susceptible to the infection.

Some of the clinical signs of FIP infection include labored breathing, enlarged abdomen, weakness or paralysis, inappetence, weight loss, a fever that comes and goes, depression, trembling, seizures, blindness, and abortion. Kittens infected with FIP virus before birth are born dead or die soon afterward. The diagnosis can be made based on the history, physical examination, and blood-work findings. Cytology examination of the fluid from the abdomen and chest can help. Tissue biopsies are occasionally required in cases that are atypical. Testing for the virus is difficult. An FIP test can be positive from a previous infection with one of those other coronaviruses, when FIP is not a problem at all.

This disease is nearly always fatal if the cat develops any of the signs described above. Some cats will respond favorably to high doses of corticosteriods that suppress the immune response caused by the virus. Developing a vaccine against this disease has been very frustrating, because the virus is difficult to grow in the laboratory and because the disease is actually caused by a hyperactive immune response to infection. Most attempts have produced a vaccine which actually gave cats FIP. Recently a vaccine has been licensed and released for use in kittens older than 16 weeks of age. It is given as drops in the nose. Since it has only been in use for a short time, the field safety and true effectiveness in reducing the death rates are unproven.

The actual disease caused by feline infectious peritonitis virus does not occur very often in most places, despite the fact that various strains of the virus are probably common. Vaccination would be important for cats in catteries with a history of FIP-related diseases, for cats that live in an area where FIP is endemic in the neighborhood cat population, or for cats whose owners want whatever protection is available to them.

Feline Leukemia Virus (FeLV)

A contagious virus transmitted between cats through saliva, urine, milk, and across the placenta, transmission takes place from fighting, sharing of food bowls and litterboxes, mutual grooming, and before birth from mother to offspring. Because transmission can take place during casual contact, one FeLV-infected cat can infect other members of a household or cattery.

Just because a cat is exposed to the virus, however, doesn't mean that he will become infected. Depending on how strong or virulent the virus strain is, it could take several weeks of exposure before an infection occurs. Most cats—about 80 percent of them—will never be exposed to enough virus to become infected.

The other 20 percent of cats will develop an initial infection. Infection begins in the tissues around the mouth and upper respiratory tract. During this early transient infection, most of these cats develop antibodies against the virus and clear it from their bodies. Those cats will be protected against further exposure from other cats. We say that they have *natural immunity* against the virus. They have essentially been vaccinated through natural exposure.

A small percentage of cats who develop an initial infection will go on to become permanently infected. Here, adequate numbers of protective antibodies are not produced. The virus spreads throughout the body and incorporates itself directly into the genetic material of the cat, especially into rapidly growing cells of the bone marrow. The virus is then continuously produced and released into the bloodstream as the bone marrow cells are also produced. This virus is detected on tests for FeLV. For a description of FeLV testing, see page 165.

Feline leukemia virus causes two different kinds of disease: cancerous and noncancerous. In a way, the virus is misnamed. Leukemia, a malignant cancer of the bone marrow, is an uncommon consequence of infection compared to the other diseases. By far and away, the virus most often causes a suppression of the bone marrow and immune system. These cats develop profoundly low red- and white-blood-cell counts; they are very, very anemic. Chronic repeated infections are common. The bacteria and viruses that cause these infections are normal inhabitants of the cat's body. Chronic respiratory and gastrointestinal diseases like sinusitis and diarrhea appear. FeLV-infected cats also develop infections with organisms that they might otherwise resist, like *Toxoplasma*, Feline Infectious Peritonitis virus, or *Haemobartonella*. Other noncancerous consequences of infection include neurologic dysfunction, abortions, stillbirths, or fading kittens that fail to survive.

Feline leukemia virus does cause cancer of the immune system. This includes most, but not all leukemias and lymphomas. Again, this is not the most common result of infection.

Feline leukemia virus can be a complicating factor in any cat illness. *It is important to test cats for the virus as part of the work-up for any serious organic, chronic, or recurrent disease*. The virus is universally fatal, usually within two years; however, this may extend for several years. During this time period repeated bouts of infection, immunosuppression, and anemia can be treated successfully, resulting in a good quality of life. Even FeLV-related cancers can be treated with chemotherapy.

It is important to isolate FeLV-positive cats from others to prevent transmission of the virus. If isolation is not possible, other cats in the household should be vaccinated. However, vaccination is not a guarantee against infection. Owners of FeLV positive cats should stay in close contact with their veterinarian. Early treatment for recurrent complications is essential to a favorable outcome.

Feline leukemia virus is not transmissible to humans. Although it has been grown in the laboratory in human-tissue culture cells, serologic testing of thousands of veterinarians has never identified an antibody against FeLV developing in humans.

Feline Lower Urinary Tract Disease (FLTD, Feline Urologic Syndrome, FUS)

A lot has been written about this problem in cats, and there is a lot of misinformation and misleading information in the lay literature, which has been spread by word-of-mouth. FLTD includes a wide range of disorders involving the bladder and urethra of cats. Bladder stones, crystals, malformations both congenital and acquired, tumors, and neurologic problems are included in this group. I will deal with the one aspect of FLTD that has been the greatest problem, FUS, separately (see page 128).

that has been the greatest problem, FUS, separately (see page 128).

Lower urinary tract disease involves the bladder and urethra. The general signs involving these organs are straining to urinate, urinating in inappropriate locations around the house, abnormal urine color such as from blood or pus, incontinence, inability to pass urine, abdominal pain, and dermatitis around the prepuce or vulva. These can occur in any age cat, depending upon the cause. Causes include infection, stones, crystals, trauma, tumors, nerve damage or degeneration, hormone disorders, diet, or unknown causes.

Diagnosis can sometimes be made based on history, physical examination, and blood and urinalysis. Urine cultures, abdominal radiographs, ultrasound examination of the bladder, and contrast-type radiographs of the bladder, are sometimes necessary. There are also special tests measuring nerve function of the bladder and urethra available at some referral hospitals. Biopsies are done and an analysis of all bladder stones is essential.

Treatment and prognosis depends upon the cause of the signs. Antibiotics are chosen based on the results of cultures and sensitivity testing. Drugs affecting bladder and urethral muscle tone can be used. Dietary management is the cornerstone of therapy for FUS, the most common form of FLTD. Dietary manipulation is also essential to the effective treatment of urinary tract stones, depending upon the type of stone. Surgery is useful in some cases to correct anatomic defects, remove stone and obtain biopsies. See also *Feline Urologic Syndrome.*

Feline Panleukopenia (feline distemper)

Although the disease caused by panleukopenia virus is called feline distemper, this virus more closely resembles parvovirus in dogs. In fact, during the initial outbreak and epidemic of the disease in the 1970s, feline panleukopenia vaccine was used to vaccinate dogs against parvovirus until a specific canine parvovirus vaccine could be developed. Think of the countless number of dog lives saved by cats!

The virus is highly contagious among all species of cats. Cats harbor the virus inside their gastrointestinal tract and shed it in their feces. The virus can live for a long time in the environment outside of the body. That means it can be tracked all around as cats move in and out of the litterbox. Panleukopenia virus is also very resistant to disinfectants. All this means is that it is very easy for susceptible cats and kittens to come in contact with the virus, ingest it, and become infected.

Panleukopenia virus has four major target organs once it enters the body: lymph nodes, the bone marrow, the inside lining of the gastrointestinal system, and the brain of kittens during late gestation. The infection of lymph nodes and bone marrow causes very low white blood cell counts and suppresses the immune system. The infection of the gastrointestinal tract wipes out the protective barrier to invasion by bacteria, allowing their passage into the bloodstream. Pregnant queens infected with panleukopenia virus may have abortions. Kittens infected just before birth will have locomotor difficulty—that is, they will have tremors, may fall over as they try to walk, and have a "bunny-hop" gait because the virus invaded the brain.

The clinical signs of panleukopenia are fever, depression, inappetence, vomiting, diarrhea, dehydration, and coma. Diagnosis is usually assumed based on the physical examination, clinical signs, and a history of inadequate vaccination. Treatment involves supportive care: intravenous fluids, injectable antibiotics, warmth, quiet, and food once the vomiting and diarrhea are under control. Severe infections, especially in very young kittens, can end in death. Kittens born with brain defects that affect their gait can learn to compensate for this disability and live a normal life.

This virus is everywhere; unvaccinated cats are very susceptible to infection. Not every cat that is exposed will become sick with the full-blown disease, but kittens and young cats are at the greatest risk. Serious panleukopenia is preventable by vaccination. Pregnant queens should receive a vaccine containing a killed form of the virus because the modified-live panleukopenia virus contained in most vaccines can infect the developing fetal brain tissue and cause birth defects much the same as the "wild-type" virus.

Feline Urologic Syndrome (FUS)

The most common FLTD is Feline Urologic Syndrome. Feline urologic syndrome results when minerals present in the urine form a crystalline, sandlike substance. This sand sits in the bladder like sand in your bathing suit. It sloshes around, irritating the inside lining of the bladder. The lining may bleed and the cat is very uncomfortable. He will have the urge to void even if there is little urine in the bladder.

These events occur in *both male and female cats*, and usually in adults. The sand mixes with proteins secreted by the bladder lining. In female cats, this material passes through the wide, short urethra. In the male, the sand-protein mixture can plug the long, narrow urethra.

There have been many attempts to blame this problem on an infectious agent like a virus or bacteria. In one or two instances, a virus has been isolated from affected cats. This virus may have been the cause or it may have been a fluke. That's

not to say that a virus might not someday be implicated. It's just that with current research, no virus has ever been proven to be the culprit. Bacteria are not the primary cause.

So far, the only factor that has been shown to be consistently involved in the development of FUS in cats is *diet*. Alkaline diets and diets high in magnesium can cause the urine to become alkaline and predispose cats to FUS. This is most often the case with supermarket and other inexpensive dry cat foods. Canned cat foods are less often involved, as the increase in water content causes more urine to be produced and the crystals to be washed out of the bladder. Obesity can contribute to the problem too. Fat, lazy cats don't go to the litterbox and void as much as they should.

Once the inflammation associated with FUS has occurred, there may be a secondary infection by bacteria. This happens in only about 2 percent of all cases! *The cystitis caused by the sand or crystals is the most common form of cystitis in cats and it is almost always sterile.* This is a very important point to understand. Antibiotics alone are not effective. *The only appropriate therapy involves dietary management.*

Treatment of FUS depends upon the severity of the signs. Simple cystitis without obstruction appears as straining to urinate, blood in the urine, or urinating in unusual locations (Many cats use the bathtub, as if to say, "Hey, look at this. . ."); it responds well to dietary management alone. Antibiotics are only appropriate if a urinalysis and culture reveal an infection. If the cat is obstructed, he will strain to urinate without producing urine. He will become depressed, inappetent, and vomit from the toxins that build up in the blood because of kidney failure. Death follows coma in about 18 hours.

In cases of urethral obstruction, a catheter must be passed into the bladder as soon as possible. Subcutaneous or intravenous fluids are given to promote the elimination of toxic waste products that have accumulated in the blood and to counteract the increased urination that follows relief of the obstruction. A urinary catheter is left in place for at least 24 hours. Once the catheter is removed, antibiotics are begun because the catheter has allowed bacteria into the bladder. Dietary management is also initiated in obstructed cats.

Initial dietary management begins with feeding a diet that dissolves the sand or crystals by making the urine more acidic. The higher salt content of this diet also induces the cat to drink a lot of water, thus increasing the amount of urine produced. This washes out the bladder. The best diet for this purpose is a prescription-type diet rather than a home-cooked one or the supplementation of a commercial diet. It is essential to keep the urine in an acidic state and increase the dietary salt intake to carefully controlled and consistent levels. This is not possible with supplements.

Once the urine appears normal on urinalysis, a maintenance diet is used to control the magnesium intake and urine acidity. Currently there is no supermarket cat food that safely achieves this goal, no matter what the label claims. There are prescription-type diets and "premium" diets that can be used. Recurrence of FUS is almost guaranteed to happen if the owner goes back to feeding commercial cat foods.

And now a word about ash. Many pet food manufacturers claim that their foods promote a healthy urinary tract and are suitable for cats with FUS because they are low in ash. Ash refers to the total mineral content of the diet, not just the magnesium. Low ash does not necessarily mean low magnesium. Magnesium levels should not exceed 20 mg/100 kcal of diet in any cat.

In the long term, urine acidity plays just as much of a role. In the laboratory, acidity is measured and reported as a term called the *pH.* Many pet-food manufacturers add acidifiers to the food to promote low urine pH (high acidity). Sometimes they add acidifiers in amounts that can cause a metabolic acidosis condition in the blood. This can result in the leaching of calcium from the bones and osteoporosis when fed over a long period of time. Overzealous use of urinary acidifiers depletes the body of potassium which has been shown to cause kidney disease in cats. The urine pH should not go below 5.8 or above 6.4 in cats. The owner should test this for themselves using test paper called *litmus paper* if they use urinary acidifiers, and specifically inquire about the pH range of the urine when commercial or prescription-type diets are fed. Litmus paper can be obtained through a pharmacy or your veterinarian.

Information about magnesium intake and urine pH is rarely on the label or available from the manufacturer. You should follow your veterinarian's recommendation regarding dietary management for the life of your cat. Change the diet only after consulting your doctor and after the manufacturer has supported all claims related to urinary tract health.

Feline Viral Rhinotracheitis

This is one of several viruses that cause upper respiratory disease. A watery to thick mucus or purulent discharge from the nose, sneezing, noisy breathing, a secondary conjunctivitis, inappetence, depression, and mild dehydration are the signs. An accumulation of dried, crusty debris can "glue" the eyelids shut, especially in kittens. In a few cases, corneal ulcers and pneumonia may be complications. The disease is much more severe in kittens than in adult cats.

Treatment involves supportive care. Although the disease involves a virus, antibiotics both oral and in the eyes are given to control the secondary bacterial infection. Since these cats can't smell their food, they won't eat. Starvation is not a part of the treatment plan, so force feeding and fluids are important.

Rhinotracheitis is not a life-threatening disease unless the kitten or cat is otherwise debilitated and treatment is delayed. It can be controlled by proper vaccination. Most infected kittens and cats will become carriers of the virus and may have periodic bouts with respiratory disease when under stress. See also *Calicivirus, Chlamydia, Conjunctivitis, Sinusitis.*

Food Allergy (food intolerance, food hypersensitivity, eosinophilic, lymphocytic, plasmacytic gastroenteritis)

Adverse reactions to foods can be caused by any substance in that food, whether it is a major ingredient such as beef, eggs, or soy, or a minor one such as dairy products, preservatives, dyes, or "fillers." Food allergies manifest themselves in one of two ways. They either cause skin problems, with severe itching, redness, sores and hair loss around the face and sometimes body, or gastroenteritis with vomiting and/or diarrhea.

Cats with food allergies are usually but not always adults. The clinical signs of food intolerance can occur immediately after eating the offending food, or several hours later. Food allergies take time to develop. Most allergic cats have been eating the offending food for some time, even years, before the signs appear.

Diagnosis of food allergies is largely a trial and error process. Scientific studies have shown that the traditional skin testing used for inhalant allergies and the more recently developed and popular blood tests for food allergies are extremely poor determinators of food allergies. Many people press to use these tests because they are simple to do. Frustrated by the disease itself and daunted by the prospect of having to do an elimination food trial for several weeks, these tests seem like a quick fix to a complex problem. They simply don't work for food allergies, and they cost a lot of money. Gastroenteritis caused by food intolerance can be suggested by biopsying the stomach, or the small or large intestine, depending upon whether or not the cat is vomiting and the character of the diarrhea.

The only way to know what foods are offending an allergic cat is to do an elimination food trial for several weeks. *Home-cooked diets are more accurate in assessing food allergies than prescription-type hypoallergenic diets.* Many prescription-type diets are made with meat meals that are contaminated with other meats besides the one on the label. Commercial hypoallergenic diets usually have more than one protein source also. Some of the protein will come from the meat and some will come from the grains. The allergenic substance is usually a protein. A proper elimination trial consists of feeding a diet formulated with a single source of protein, preferably one that the cat has not been exposed to previously. Lamb, rabbit, venison, and horsemeat are used. Carbohydrates are usually supplied by rice which is not only easily digestible, but also contains the least amount of protein of all the grains used for energy. Other hypoallergenic diets use tofu, mashed potatoes, green beans, fish, etc. Dietary fiber is used in moderate amounts.

A food trial using a specific diet is performed for several weeks. Initially the clinical signs may worsen or just stay the same, making everyone involved discouraged. Several different diets may be needed before a truly hypoallergenic diet is found. Once the clinical signs have been resolved, other foods may be added one at a time.

If food trials alone are not effective in eliminating the gastrointestinal signs of food intolerance, anti-inflammatory drugs and medication to suppress the immune response are used. If an allergic cat responds well to a food trial, a balanced prescription-type hypoallergenic diet may be introduced, or the owner may be forced to feed a home-cooked diet with fat, vitamin, and mineral supplements for the rest of the cat's life. The diets used for food trials are never complete or balanced for long term feeding. Drug therapy may also continue indefinitely, or gradually be withdrawn.

The prognosis is good despite the possibility that the cat might develop an allergy to the hypoallergenic diet with time.

G

Gastroenteritis (vomiting and/or diarrhea)

Vomiting and diarrhea prompt a lot of phone calls to veterinary hospitals, probably more so for dog owners than cat owners. Cats vomit a lot anyway. Hairballs, nondigestible remnants of a mouse carcass, parts of your houseplants show up in the darndest places and at the most inopportune times. Certain brands or flavors of foods induce vomiting (or diarrhea) in some cats. This could be from an abrupt change in diet disrupting the normal "ecology" of the gastrointestinal system, or from one of the main ingredients, preservatives, additives, or dyes used in some pet foods. Unlike dogs, cats don't often eat inanimate objects like socks or

small toys, but they do raid the trash and eat rancid chicken bones and other leftovers if they're hungry enough. And cats don't ask for a health certificate before devouring a bird. If the cat caught it, it might have been too sick to escape.

Episodes of diarrhea are a little more difficult to discover unless the cat uses a litterbox. Defecation in inappropriate places or fecal soiling of the fur around the perineum are two signs if direct observation isn't possible. Any of the above causes of vomiting can also cause diarrhea alone or in conjunction with vomiting. Intestinal parasites, bacteria, or viruses cause these signs in young animals with immature immune systems.

Acute minor vomiting and diarrhea can escalate. Botulism or other food or chemical poisonings can cause kidney or liver failure, and both include vomiting and diarrhea as part of the clinical picture. The stomach or intestines can leak or rupture if a bone becomes lodged. Heavy parasite infections, and viral and bacterial diseases in kittens can begin suddenly and progress to intractable gastroenteritis, severe dehydration, and rapid decline.

Acute minor cases can become chronic. It's important to take note of vomiting and diarrhea and watch for unexplainable, intermittent episodes that signal a potentially substantial underlying organic problem. Diabetes and hyperthyroidism are examples of serious illnesses that may initially begin with intermittent low-grade gastroenteritis.

Most acute cases of vomiting and diarrhea are minor and self-limiting; they resolve on their own without any treatment. These cats act fairly normally, avoid food for a day or so, or may continue to eat. Again, repeated episodes of vomiting and diarrhea should be investigated, especially if there are changes in water intake, urination, body weight, or behavior.

Causes of severe or chronic gastroenteritis are determined based on the history of the illness; physical examination; and blood, urine, and fecal analysis. A veterinarian might need several diagnostic tools: radiology, endoscopy, exploratory, ultrasonography, cytology, or biopsy before a definitive diagnosis is made. Sometimes a trial-and-error approach, combining treatment with diagnosis using a course of antibiotics, anthelmintics, or dietary trial, is necessary.

Treatment depends upon the cause (or suspected cause). This can include drugs, surgery, and supportive care. Dietary management is almost always an important part of treatment. The cat with an upset stomach does this on his own when he stops eating for a day. Dietary management usually means withholding food and/or water so the gastrointestinal tract can rest and begin to heal. When the protective barrier to the stomach or intestine is damaged by toxins or bacteria, food substances can cross and trigger the body's immune system and cause an allergic-type reaction. This can make the vomiting or diarrhea worse and can sensitize the cat to food allergies in the future. Dietary management involves feeding a highly digestible, carbohydrate-based diet with a single source of high-quality protein, low in fat and low to moderate in the amount of fiber. Some diarrheas respond to higher fiber diets than others. Both homecooked and prescription diets are used.

H

Haemobartonella
See *Feline Infectious Anemia*.

Hairballs
The medical term for hairballs is *trichobezoar*. This is an accumulation of hair inside the stomach. Hairballs develop because cats don't have what we call "housekeeping functions." That is, their stomach does not contract and empty in between meals. Cats also have a very small *pylorus*, or outflow opening to their stomach, making it difficult to pass large quantities of hair that might accumulate after grooming, especially in long-haired breeds. So if my cat Cocoa curls up in a patch of sunshine and takes a nice bath, the hair he consumes will either have to pass through with his next meal, or

come back up the same way it went down. And you know how that is, you're either fast asleep and wake to hear the cat making that hairball-sort-of-retching-sound on the quilt at the foot of your bed, or else your bare foot finds the cold, wet pelage in the morning.

An occasional hairball is not of concern, but chronic vomiting due to hairballs can be a problem. There are several remedies. Laxatives containing flavored petrolatum are given once or twice a week. This is a sort of hit or miss therapy; the cat may or may not have a hairball at the time you give a dose of laxative. The petrolatum helps the hair to slide through the pylorus. The better method for hairball control is to feed a canned diet high in fiber. The fiber traps the hair and drags it out of the pylorus. Feeding even a small portion of the daily diet as a fiber diet can keep the stomach clear of hair and reduce the frequency of vomiting.

Hyperthyroidism

This is a condition caused by excessive levels of thyroid hormone in the blood. The excess hormone is produced by a tumor in the thyroid glands which are normally located in the superficial tissues in the neck. The tumors are usually (but not always) benign; that is, they do not spread or metastasize to other tissues. They can, however, grow to a large size and cause the gland to drop lower in the neck or just inside the thorax. A small percentage of the tumors are malignant but, this can only be determined by obtaining a biopsy.

This is a disease mostly in older cats. The tumors develop in one or both of the glands. Some cats will develop a tumor in one gland and then sometime later develop one in the other gland. The excess hormone exerts a number of effects on the cat to cause the clinical signs. The hallmark signs of a hyperthyroid cat are weight loss in the face of a ravenous appetite, restlessness, excessive water intake, and urination. Hyperthyroid cats are often very difficult to handle. They may have intermittent soft, smelly, and voluminous stools.

The excess thyroid hormone has other effects too. It causes a type of heart disease called hypertrophic cardiomyopathy and an extremely rapid heart rate. There may be effects on the liver. Because these cats are usually old, other diseases can be present, like kidney disease or other tumors.

Hyperthyroid cats are some of the skinniest cats I've ever seen. It can take months or years for the excess hormone to cause all the effects mentioned above. The hormone levels don't have to be that high to cause these effects, either— sometimes they're just at the upper end of the normal range.

The diagnosis is made by the history reported by the owner, physical examination findings, especially the presence of a palpable tumor in the neck, and blood tests for thyroid hormone. A thorough evaluation of the blood must be made along with radiographs of the chest and an EKG.

There are several forms of treatment. There are drugs that work to lower the level of hormone in the blood. These drugs can have some very serious side effects, especially on the bone marrow and liver. They must be given one to three times a day, which can be quite difficult in a fractious cat with heart disease! Some cats become refractory to the drugs after a while so they don't work anymore. The medications have to be given for the rest of the cat's life, which can be considerable. My cat Willie developed a thyroid tumor at the relatively young age of twelve.

Another alternative is surgical removal of the gland with the tumor. This is curative; that is, once you remove the gland, the problem goes away and you don't have to deal with it anymore. There are risks though, because these cats have a greater risk of complications (including death) under anesthesia. It is customary to give cats medication to lower the thyroid levels and stabilize the heart for several weeks prior to surgery in order to decrease this risk. Once some of the clinical signs of hyperthyroidism abate, surgery is performed. Unlike the two other treatment programs, the tissue that is recovered during surgery is available to be examined for malignancy.

Another surgical complication relates to calcium. Closely associated with each thyroid gland is another pair of tiny glands called parathyroid glands. These are responsible for regulating the amount of calcium in the body. Because of the close association with the thyroids, these glands are invariably damaged or unavoidably removed when the affected thyroid is removed. This is not a problem if only one thyroid contains a tumor because there is an untouched pair on the other side. If both thyroids are tumorous, all four parathyroid glands may be damaged. As a result, they may cease to produce the hormone needed to keep the body's calcium level up to normal. Low blood calcium can have significant effects on the heart, muscle, and nervous tissue, causing seizures or dangerously low heart rates. Most of the time this is a temporary side effect, but it does mean that calcium supplements must be given until the parathyroid glands recover.

A third complication of surgery relates to the location of the tumorous gland. Most can be felt within the neck area unless the tumor has dropped into the chest cavity. To confirm the location, a low-level radioactive isotope that will be taken up by the tumor is given by injection. A special camera is used to take a picture to locate it. This must be done at a special referral hospital (see below). The surgery to remove tumors in this area is much more complicated and the anesthesia is tricky.

The third option for treatment involves an injection of a radioactive isotope of iodine, an integral element in the chemical makeup of thyroid hormone. The radioactive iodine is selectively taken up by the glands, which are destroyed by the radioactive emissions, just like other radiation therapies for cancers. The best thing about this treatment is that only the thyroid glands are affected, unlike conventional radiation treatments. No anesthesia is required and the parathyroid glands are preserved. Most of the time only one treatment is needed.

I[131] treatment, as it is called, is only available at referral medical centers because a special license is required to handle and dispose of radioactive substances. There are only a few hospitals equipped to perform this procedure, so it may not be accessible. It also means that your cat must be hospitalized for some period of time. Once the cat has received the injection, all the feces and urine must be collected and disposed of according to federal guidelines. The cat cannot be discharged from the hospital until the radioactive emissions emanating from the cat are below a strict level. The cat would be the hot stuff he thinks he is.

After all this, I'm sure you're wondering why anyone would treat a cat for hyperthyroidism given that there are probably other geriatric diseases going on at the same time, the complications are formidable, and the expense sizable. To put all this into perspective, most affected cats have one or two readily palpable tumors that can safely be removed by surgery. Modern anesthetics minimize the risks, provided the cat is stabilized by medication for several weeks ahead of time. I have done this surgery in many eighteen-year-old cats. Once treated, the side effects of the excessive hormone go away. Without treatment, the cat's quality of life and general physical condition are poor.

I

Incontinence

An inability to control urination voluntarily is defined as *urinary incontinence.* Cats with this condition will dribble urine. They may do so constantly or intermittently as the bladder achieves a certain degree of fullness. They may leak urine only when lying down or during sleep. The corresponding inability to control the passage of feces is termed *fecal incontinence*. These cats will involuntarily drop feces from the rectum due to lack of anal sphincter tone.

Incontinence results from anatomic, neurologic, endocrine, traumatic, degenerative, and infectious causes. In feline medicine, one of the most common instances of incontinence occurs in association with the tailless trait in Manx cats. Atypical development of the last few vertebrae and the nerves controlling urination and colon function often results in both urinary and fecal incontinence (or constipation) in members of this breed.

Tail injuries are also frequently associated with urinary and fecal incontinence. Cats who get their tail trapped under tires or feet, closed into doors, or yanked by small children suffer from dislocation of the spinal vertebrae and dislocation of the associated nerves that innervate the bladder and colon. Incontinence can be temporary or permanent. Frequently the tail must be amputated due to loss of innervation.

Severe urinary tract infections, bladder stones, severe or chronic diarrhea, spinal nerve degeneration, and infections and tumors are a few other conditions associated with incontinence. Urinary incontinence itself can lead to chronic bladder infections, so it is very important to determine which came first in that situation. Incontinent cats will have a chronic dermatitis around the perineum and along the inside of the rear legs from the scalding of the urine and feces dribbling down the skin. This is painful and irritating to the cat who then licks and cleans himself, creating an even worse dermatitis.

Treatment for incontinence depends upon the cause. Neurologic testing to identify a primary nerve problem to the bladder is available at several teaching hospitals; however most veterinarians rely on the history, physical examination findings, blood, urine and fecal examination, radiographs, and endoscopy to identify the cause and decide on an appropriate course of therapy. There are several drugs that can be used to affect the bladder and urethral sphincter tone. Incontinence related to trauma may resolve with time.

Internal Parasites

Parasites infect almost every tissue or organ system of the body. Only a few are of major clinical significance in the cat: *gastrointestinal, respiratory, and circulatory*. Internal parasites are sometimes detected through direct observation of worms in the stool or vomitus, or in the case of some tapeworms, by observing the segments crawling on the fur around the anus. More commonly, they must be detected by examination of the feces for eggs or other stages of the parasite's life cycle.

Internal parasites don't always cause disease. Some are "well-adapted" to their host, which is advantageous to the parasite too. Parasites are more likely to infect younger animals because their immune system is immature. As an animal matures, the immune system makes them more resistant to infection in the first place. The immune system is likely to clear up infections in adult animals, so that many cats are probably infected but never show clinical signs of disease because the parasite is kept in check and eventually eliminated.

Parasite damage results from any stage in the organism's life cycle. Internal parasites cause disease in a number of ways. They obstruct organs, compete for nutrients, destroy tissue by feeding, migrating and disrupting normal architecture, and incite inflammation. Parasites weaken young kittens and make them more susceptible to secondary illnesses and infection. I will discuss the more common parasites found in cats. Keep in mind that there are others.

Gastrointestinal parasites are the most important of the internal parasites in cats. Of these, two species of *roundworms* with similar life cycles are the greatest plague. Adult roundworms of both species live in the cat's intestines and produce eggs which exit with the feces. Soil or litter becomes contaminated with eggs that another cat ingests when it licks its paws. Once inside the cat, the eggs hatch out tiny larvae that penetrate the tissues of the intestine and start migrating through the liver, lungs, and muscle tissue of the cat.

All the while they are traveling through the tissues they are developing through stages of maturation. Eventually, the larvae find their way back into the intestine where they grow up into adult worms and begin to produce eggs on their own. Anthelmintic or worm medication kill these adult worms in the intestinal tract.

That would be the end of the story if it were not for the wayward larvae that never make it back into the intestinal tract but stay in the body tissues. In male cats, that's the end of the line for them. But for female cats, those larvae cross the mammary glands into the milk, infecting the nursing kittens. Once inside the tissues of the kittens, they go on to find their way into the kitten's digestive tract so that several weeks after birth, the kittens can have huge numbers of long, spaghetti-like worms obstructing their intestines and causing a pot-bellied appearance, vomiting, diarrhea, and malnutrition.

There is no drug that will kill the larvae as they migrate through tissues. That's why it is extremely difficult to eliminate these intestinal parasites from cats. Kittens are not born with the fully developed adult worms. It takes about nine weeks for the larvae to find their way into the intestinal tract and to begin to produce eggs that can be detected on a fecal examination. Your kitten's feces should be examined for parasite eggs no earlier than at nine weeks of age. It may take several stool sample evaluations to completely eliminate the possibility of intestinal worms.

Two other less common intestinal parasites are *hookworms* and *whipworms*. Both worms attach themselves to the lining of the intestinal tract and suck blood. Diarrhea and weight loss are the most significant consequences. Adult worms produce eggs that are passed in the feces. Cats acquire these infections by ingesting the larvae from these worms. There are anthelmintic medicines that kill the adult parasites.

Two types of *tapeworms* live in the intestinal tract of cats. Cats don't mind, but their owners do. *Dipylidium*, or the *flea tapeworm* looks like moving pieces of rice around the perineum or worse, on the owner after holding the cat. Inside the cat, these are actually flat, linked segments shaped like melon seeds. The tapeworm breaks apart into individual segments and chains of segments that exit with the feces. Each segment contains packets of tapeworm eggs. The segments dry up and are eaten by flea larvae. The eggs remain inside the flea larva as it matures into an adult flea. When the cat eats the flea while grooming, the eggs are liberated and a new tapeworm grows and the life cycle is completed. The only way to rid a cat of flea tapeworms is to control the flea life cycle too.

The other type of tapeworm infects cats that hunt. *Taenia* tapeworms are long and flat. The segments don't pass in the feces very often; instead the segments rupture and release the eggs while still inside the intestinal tract. They can be detected in routine fecal flotation tests. The eggs are deposited in the soil and consumed by small mammals like mice or rats. The eggs hatch in the mouse or rat. When a cat hunts and eats the mouse, the tapeworm completes its lifecycle.

Another common intestinal parasite in cats are *Coccidia*, which are not worms, but a group of one-celled organisms in the Protozoa family. These parasites are easily transmitted through the consumption of eggs called cysts that are passed in feces of infected animals. The cysts hatch to produce the coccidia organisms that reproduce in the small intestine. Many kittens and adult cats harbor these parasites without any signs. Others will develop diarrhea containing fresh blood. In order to avoid future problems, most veterinarians treat coccidiosis, even if it isn't causing any problem, at the time it is detected.

Toxoplasma is one of the most important parasites in the coccidia group. The parasite is a "two host" parasite like the *Taenia* tapeworm. The primary host is the cat who harbors the adult organisms in the intestinal tract. *Toxoplasma* rarely causes disease in cats. Some cats will develop a mild, transient case of diarrhea, but most will have no signs of infection. In a cat whose immune system is compromised by another illness, such as a feline leukemia virus infection, *Toxoplasma* may cause severe diarrhea and wasting.

The mature form of the parasite is a cyst that passes with the feces. The cysts must mature in the soil or litterbox for 48 hours before they can infect the secondary host. (We call these "infective cysts.") In the normal course of things, the secondary host is a small rodent, like a mouse or a rat. This host consumes infective cysts that contaminate its paws when it walks through soil containing cat feces. Once inside the secondary host, the cysts develop into the next stage in the parasite's life cycle, zoites. Zoites cross the wall of the intestine and enter the blood where they travel and become encysted throughout the tissues of the secondary host. When a cat kills and eats the secondary host, i.e., a mouse, it consumes the encysted zoites with the flesh. Digestion releases them to mature into the form that is passed in the feces. *Toxoplasma* can only complete its life cycle inside a cat.

Toxoplasma infections are a concern not so much because of what the parasite does inside the cat, because it rarely causes a problem, but because of the problems that develop in the secondary host. Cattle, sheep, goats, and other herbivorous animals accidentally ingest the infective cysts while grazing on land that is used by cats for elimination. Dogs ingest the zoites if they hunt small herbivorous prey like mice. The zoites don't go on to mature in the intestines of these animals as they do in the cat, but rather encyst in the muscle, and udders, or mammary tissues. The zoite forms of the *Toxoplasma* parasite cause signs of the flu.

Humans become infected with zoites, too. People can consume the infective cysts directly just like cattle, if they don't wear gloves while working in a garden where cats defecate. People take in encysted zoites when they eat undercooked beef or, as in some cultures, drink unpasteurized milk. This is particularly a problem for pregnant women. The zoite has an affinity for encysting in the brain tissue of the developing fetus. Animals and babies may be born with tragic birth defects.

Toxoplasma is usually an incidental finding in fecal flotation tests. A blood test is available to determine if a cat has ever been infected with *Toxoplasma*; however, a positive test does not indicate an active infection. This is important to remember. Some physicians will advise pregnant women to have their cats tested for *Toxoplasma*, and recommend that cats testing positive be removed from the household. Likewise, a negative fecal flotation test does not eliminate the possibility that a cat is a carrier, since the organisms may be shed intermittently and in low numbers and therefore be difficult to detect.

To reiterate, the only way to confirm an active case of *Toxoplasma* in cats is by finding the parasite in the feces. The only way to protect yourself against *Toxoplasma* infection is to avoid eating undercooked beef, lamb, and unpasteurized milk. Always wear gloves while working in the garden. Cysts become capable of infection 48 hours after defecation. Remove feces from the litterbox within 24 hours.

Toxoplasmosis is rarely treated. Combinations of antibiotics are sometimes used.

Another major protozoal-type parasite of significance in cats is *Giardia*. Cats probably acquire the infection by drinking water contaminated by feces containing cysts. The cysts mature into zoites in the small intestine. Most cats do not have any signs of infection. A few cats get diarrhea that can be watery or soft, gray, and very foul-smelling. The parasite prevents digestion and absorption of nutrients. *Giardia* can be seen on direct smears made from diarrheic feces. The cysts can be detected on flotation and with special tests of fresh feces. Do not refrigerate fecal samples that are to be tested for *Giardia*. All cats testing positive for *Giardia* should be treated.

Some of these parasites can be transmitted to humans. These are called *zoonotic* parasites. Children are at the greatest risk because of their hygiene practices and immature immune systems. Children consuming roundworm eggs can develop *visceral larval migrans* as the larva migrate in their tissues. Hookworm larvae penetrate the skin to cause a rash called *cutaneous larval migrans* in children who walk barefoot over ground contaminated with the larvae that have hatched from the eggs. Some tapeworms undergo part of their life cycle in humans, including the flea tapeworm. There is some evidence that the *Giardia* species found in animals will also infect people.

There are two important **respiratory system parasites** of cats. *Paragonimus* is a fluke that lives in the lungs. The fluke creates a cystic space in the tissue and releases eggs which are coughed up and swallowed and then exit in the feces. Snails and crayfish feeding on dung and rotting debris eat the fluke eggs. The eggs hatch and grow inside the mollusk or crustacean. Cats preying on these animals eat the developing fluke which is released by digestion into the cat's gastrointestinal tract. It migrates to the lungs where it feeds on lung tissue and body fluids, causing intense inflammation. *Paragonimus* infections cause cough, weight loss, lack of appetite, pneumonia, and sometimes fever.

The diagnosis is made by detecting the fluke eggs on a fecal flotation test and by observing the masslike cysts on chest radiographs. The changes seen on the radiographs look similar to those seen with other diseases like lung cancer and pneumonia caused by fungus, so these must be ruled out as well in cats being evaluated for cough.

These cats should have blood tests and follow-up radiographs done to properly monitor treatment which includes anthelminthic drugs, antibiotics for pneumonia, and supportive care if necessary.

The other lung parasite infecting cats is a tiny worm called *Aelurostrongylus* that lives in the airways and causes pneumonia. The worms lay eggs that hatch into larvae while still inside the lungs. The larvae crawl up the airways, and are swallowed and excreted with feces. The larvae are then eaten by snails who are in turn eaten by mice who are in turn eaten by. . . and become infected. The diagnosis is made by finding the larvae in samples from a bronchial wash or Baerman fecal analysis (see Glossary).

Only a few cats will develop severe pneumonia. The cat's immune system usually clears up the infection on its own. Severe infections are treated the same as other parasitic pneumonias.

There is one clinically significant **circulatory system parasite**. *Dirofilariasis*, or *heartworm disease*, has historically only been considered a problem for dogs. In recent years, more and more heartworm-infected cats have also been diagnosed in areas where heartworm disease incidence in dogs is high. Heartworms live in the arteries that exit the heart and carry blood to the lungs for oxygen. They cause obstruction of the blood flow and severe inflammation in the walls of the arteries. The adult heartworms release offspring called *microfilaria* into the bloodstream. The infective larvae are transmitted between animals by mosquitoes. Within six months, they have developed into more adult heartworms.

After a few months to years of living in the arteries, heartworms cause severe heart failure. Until then, animals remain nearly free of clinical signs. Cats may have intermittent fever, vomiting, or some breathing difficulty. Heartworm-infected cats or dogs can be asymptomatic and suddenly die. Because of the occult nature of heartworm disease and because the signs are so nonspecific, sick cats should be tested for heartworm if they live in an area where the disease is common in dogs. Heartworm-positive cats should have a complete work-up including blood evaluation, chest radiographs, and electrocardiogram prior to treatment.

Treatment depends on the degree of heart failure. Several injections of an arsenic-containing compound must be given to kill the adults. Complications as a result of the treatment are common. If clinical signs of heart failure are also present, these must also be addressed.

Some veterinarians use heartworm preventive medications in cats if they are at risk. Confining cats (and dogs) indoors to eliminate exposure to mosquitoes is only effective if you can confine the mosquitoes outdoors! Some people have insisted that their animals are not at risk for heartworm because "they stay in their own yard." This, of course, is preposterous.

K

Kidney Disease

Together with the liver, the kidneys are responsible for filtering waste products and toxins from the blood. Kidneys regulate the acidity, blood pressure, number of red cells, and the concentration of salts in the blood. Because the kidneys have such a tremendously pivotal role in maintaining the body's "balance" or *homeostasis*, diseases of the kidney have far-reaching effects on every other organ system: the heart, skeleton, brain, muscle, etc.

Just as with any other organ or tissue, many bacteria and viruses (such as FIP) infect the kidneys. Direct trauma (car accidents), poisons (antifreeze, ibuprofen), bacterial toxins, and kidney stones directly destroy tissue or interfere with func-

tion. The immune system can destroy the kidneys during the normal process of inflammation and immune response. Cancers grow from the kidneys, or after being transplanted there by way of the blood. There are birth defects. Persian cats and related breeds are predisposed to polycystic disease, a congenital condition where the normal kidney architecture is disrupted by many cysts, some of which can be so large as to leave only a remnant of the outer surface tissue.

Chronic renal or kidney disease is the most common kidney disease in cats and is the most common cause of nontraumatic death in geriatric cats. The cause is rarely known. The kidneys are damaged by infection or toxins or simply deteriorate with age. Early in the course of the disease, the healthy remaining tissue manages to carry the workload quite well. Most cats live normally until 75 percent of their kidney function is lost. This can take months to years after the initial insult. That's why we rarely know what initiated the problem at the time of diagnosis—the cat has been healthy with no signs of any kidney problems at all.

A cat can develop kidney disease at any age. Chronic renal disease is usually seen in middle-aged to older cats. It can be asymptomatic, as I have said. It is one of those diseases that veterinarians look for in presurgical lab work. Clinical signs include weight loss, inappetence, pallor, vomiting, diarrhea, increased water consumption (polydipsia) and urination (polyuria), dehydration, weakness, and in the later stages, depression, seizures, bleeding disorders, and coma.

Notice that these are all nonspecific signs of illness. Laboratory tests help to confirm the diagnosis, but keep in mind that the test results are likely to be normal until 75 percent of the kidney function is lost. A complete blood count, chemistry panel, analysis and culture of the urine are done. Radiographs of the abdomen and ultrasound examination check for stones and assess kidney size and shape. A biopsy is essential if cancer is suspected. A biopsy often gets closer to the cause and helps the veterinarian to decide on a treatment plan and prognosis, especially if the veterinarian thinks that poisoning or an ongoing insult is possible.

Treatment for renal disease is aimed at supporting the remaining kidney function and correcting the effects of kidney disease on other systems in the body. Fluids, either intravenous or subcutaneous, are the mainstay of therapy. We push the fluids in high volume to help wash out the accumulating toxins in a process called *diuresis.* Antiemetics control vomiting and antiulcer drugs control the gastritis associated with kidney disease and improve the filtering capacity of the healthy remaining tissue. Renal dis-

ease has profound effects on the skeleton, causing a leaching of calcium and phosphorus from bones. Drugs and diet are used to lower the blood-phosphorus levels to control this process.

An important complication of renal disease is anemia. The healthy kidney secretes the hormone *erythropoietin* that acts on the bone marrow to stimulate the production of red blood cells. If the kidneys are diseased, erythropoietin may not be produced and the cat in turn becomes anemic. Erythropoietin can now be made in the laboratory and is available commercially for treatment of anemias associated with renal failure. It is a very expensive drug, but worth the cost because it works. Experience is showing that cats seem to feel better, manage better, and possibly live longer with chronic kidney disease if the anemia can be corrected.

Dietary management is important in renal-disease patients. The diet should be low in phosphorus. This is so important that drugs are sometimes used to decrease the absorption of phosphorus in conjunction with low-phosphorus diets. Low-phosphorus diets are usually lower in protein, too. By lowering the protein in the diet there is less nitrogen waste product for the handicapped kidneys to excrete and patients usually feel better if they're eating a lower protein diet. There is some scientific evidence to suggest that lower protein and phosphorus diets may slow down the progression of the kidney disease, although this is highly controversial.

Cats with kidney disease often have low-serum potassium levels. Dietary management includes supplementing the diet with potassium by feeding a diet higher in potassium as some prescription-type diets provide. Liquid potassium supplements are also available. Follow your veterinarian's instructions when using liquid potassium supplements and measure carefully. Excessive potassium supplementation can lead to rapid heart failure and death.

There are several problems with low-protein diets, potassium supplements, and cats, the most important of which is that they aren't very palatable. Kidney-disease patients usually have a poor appetite anyway. Add to that a cat's finicky eating habits and you've got a lethal combination. Renal disease patients must eat. This is the biggest prognostic factor for kidney disease in cats. All the fluids and drugs in the world are not going to turn the patient around if he won't eat. Initially, force-feeding by hand or tube can be done while the other treatments have time to work, but eventually the cat must eat on his own.

The prognosis for kidney disease is variable. Acute infections, trauma, stones, and toxins carry a good prognosis if the damage is not extensive and ongoing. Even clinical chronic renal disease can have a good prognosis if it is managed early and well. Many older cats with chronic renal disease do very well even if they need frequent subcutaneous fluid therapy at home. Renal cancers are poorly responsive to chemotherapy but surgical removal of a cancerous kidney before the cancer spreads can be curative. Polycystic disease and other congenital kidney disorders usually have a poor prognosis, resulting in early death or euthanasia. Ultimately, the outcome will depend upon how much healthy kidney tissue is present and how many other organ systems are also affected.

L

Leukemia

Leukemia is a cancer in which malignant cells multiply in the bloodstream and bone marrow. Like its soft-tissue counterpart lymphoma, leukemias are usually caused by feline leukemia virus, although this is not the most common consequence of the infection.

Malignant leukemia cells obliterate the bone marrow, replacing the normal blood-element forming tissue. These cats are profoundly anemic, have few normal white blood cells to fight infection, and limited numbers of platelets for blood clotting. Leukemic cats are pale, weak, inappetent, and may have a fever. They usually test positive for FeLV.

Leukemia is treated with chemotherapeutic drugs. It is not as responsive as lymphoma, although there are some newer experimental drugs being tested. See also *Lymphoma, Cancer*.

Linear Foreign Body

Used within the context of a sentence, this disease would be: Your cat has a linear foreign body, which means he's swallowed a thread or piece of string. This is fairly obvious if the thread is wrapped around the base of the tongue as they often are or, in the case of my cat Willie, if you happen to notice the colorful extra "tail" that hangs from the rectum. Willie got into my knitting when she was a kitten and ate a piece of green yarn.

Linear foreign body is not easy to diagnose if it doesn't appear at either end of the cat. The doctor can sometimes feel the intestine

A well-organized in-house diagnostic laboratory is efficient and produces accurate laboratory results.

bunch up or in medical terms, plicate around the string. Routine radiographs or an upper GI series may identify a linear foreign body.

This is a dangerous situation for the cat. The movement of the string in the esophagus or intestine acts like a saw, cutting it open and leaking the contents into the chest or abdomen. Complications of lacerations like this include tremendous infections and scarring. Linear foreign bodies must be removed by surgery. Never pull on a string hanging from either end of your cat. Prognosis is good if laceration and infection have not occurred.

Liver Disease

Diseases involving the liver are fairly common in cats. There are four major types; I will briefly review each one. Obese cats that stop eating for some reason are prone to a disorder called *fatty liver syndrome.* The exact reason for this is not entirely understood, but it is probably triggered by the starvation process. The cat's metabolism moves fat from storage into the liver where it will be processed for energy. Once in the liver, rather than being burned for energy, the fat stays there. Fat builds up, disrupting the normal architecture of the liver so that it can no longer do its job. The fat also obstructs the flow of bile and causes the cat to become icteric or jaundiced.

Cats with fatty liver syndrome are often fat cats with a recent history of anorexia. The anorexia might be from another illness that puts the cat off food for a few days, a change in diet to which the cat objects, a change in environment such as boarding, etc. That's why cats should not go more than 48 hours without food. Fatty liver syndrome causes depression and icterus. Regardless of the initiating cause of anorexia, these cats now refuse food because of the liver disease. If the liver disease goes on long enough, the cat loses weight and muscle.

Cholangiohepatitis is another of the most common forms of liver disease. This is a severe inflammation of the liver tissue and bile duct system. There is no specific cause, although bacterial infection or some type of toxin are often implicated.

A third common type of liver disease is that which is caused by the *Feline Infectious Peritonitis virus.* This virus is discussed separately (see page 123). The hallmark sign of liver disease caused by the FIP virus is ascites, or fluid in the abdomen, although this condition can occur with other illnesses also.

The fourth most common cause of liver disease in cats is *neoplasia* or cancer. Most primary liver cancers in cats are malignant carcinomas. Caught early before metastasis and confined to only a portion of the liver, these tumors may be treated by removing the cancerous liver lobe. Secondary cancers like lymphosarcomas involving the liver have a better prognosis because they can respond to chemotherapy.

The diagnosis of liver disease is made by physical examination and blood tests, including a complete blood count, chemistry panels, and serum bile acid tests. Radiographs of the abdomen and chest are essential to determining the extent of illness. Ultrasound is used to evaluate the liver itself. A definitive diagnosis requires a biopsy or cytology. This aids not only in identifying the exact form of liver disease present, but also helps the doctor to decide what treatments will be required.

Treatment for liver disease depends on the cause. The cornerstone of treatment for fatty liver syndrome is food. These cats must be forcefed *adequate amounts* of calories. (A few fingerfuls of food won't do it; tube-feeding is required.) Fluids to correct hydration and antibiotics in combination are needed for infection. Other drugs may be dictated based on the results of the biopsy.

The prognosis for liver disease in cats has improved somewhat over the last few years, although FIP-related liver disease continues to be almost universally fatal. Most cancers of the liver are also. Chance for recovery from the more common liver diseases of fatty liver syndrome and cholangiohepatitis is much more encouraging with early diagnosis and aggressive treatment. Home treatment is ideal for cats with liver disease because of the long convalescence.

Lymphoma (malignant lymphoma)

Lymphoma is a cancer of the immune system cell called a *lymphocyte.* Lymphocytes make antibodies and assist other immune system cells to seek out, eat, and destroy bacteria, viruses, altered or abnormal cells, and foreign-tissue transplants. Lymphocytes are distributed throughout all tissues of the body, but they are concentrated like sentry guards in nodes—lymph nodes—and other similar structures near major points of entry into the body. Clusters of lymph nodes are superficially located in the neck below the ears, in front of the shoulders, under the forelegs and hindlegs, and behind the knees. Deeper lymph nodes nestle around the heart and gastrointestinal tract. Lymphocytes travel between locations in the blood and lymph vessels, stopping along the way in the spleen, liver, bone marrow, intestinal tract or anywhere they happen to be needed.

Because lymphocytes are so well distributed, lymphoma can occur anywhere within the body. This is a malignant cancer; it has usually spread by the time it's detected. Cancerous lymphocytes break away and move along by normal means to other sites where they invade, multiply, and obliterate normal tissues and organs.

Lymphoma is one of the cancers caused by feline leukemia virus, although FeLV cannot be detected in all cases. There may be other viruses, perhaps FIV, involved in those tumors. Because FeLV can infect a cat of any age, lymphoma can occur at any age.

Lymphoma cats have a varied presentation. Anorexia, chronic vomiting and diarrhea, pallor, jaundice, breathing problems, and weakness are common. The superficial lymph nodes, liver, or spleen may be prominently enlarged. If so, the diagnosis is easily made by fine needle aspiration and cytology, or biopsy. Laboratory blood tests, radiographs of the chest and abdomen, and bone marrow analysis are used to determine the spread of the disease. If there are no prominent external or abdominal lymph nodes, aspiration or biopsy must be made of other suspicious masses or fluids, to look for malignant lymphocytes.

Lymphoma is treatable with chemotherapy. Most lymphomas, with the notable exception of lymphoma in the kidneys, respond to chemotherapy drugs. Cancers that disappear with chemotherapy are said to go into *remission.* On average, lymphoma will go quickly into remission that will last about eight months. Some remissions last for shorter times, some last for longer. Patients who come out of remission can sometimes be "rescued" with other anticancer drugs that put them back into remission.

It is important to know all the tissues that have been invaded by the cancer prior to beginning chemotherapy, so that the doctor will be sure when remission has been achieved. After that, the cat is checked regularly for the cancer's return. Lymphoma is considered cured if the remission lasts for two years.

An average of eight months may not seem like very long, but in proportion to the entire cat's life, eight months is significant. It's time spent adjusting to the idea of losing a cherished pet. The cost for lymphoma chemotherapy is not very great and there are minimal side effects. See also *Leukemia, Cancer*.

M

Miliary Dermatitis (scabby cat disease)

With scabs or crusts occurring over most of the cat's body, miliary dermatitis is most often caused by fleas. Not necessarily from a severe infestation, the scabs erupt from a hypersensitivity to the flea saliva. These cats are usually intensely itchy. A secondary bacterial skin infection can result from the self-trauma of scratching.

Other things can cause miliary dermatitis: food intolerance and generalized ringworm infections are two. Skin scrapings, cultures, and biopsies may be required to deter-mine the exact cause(s). Treatment will depend upon the results of the laboratory tests. Flea control is essential. Corticosteroids, antibiotics, antifungal medications, and food trials may be necessary.

O

Otitis

Otitis refers to an inflammation of the ear. *Otitis externa* is an inflammation of the ear flap or *pinna* and the canal, and is the most frequently diagnosed type of otitis in cats. When the inflammation extends past the eardrum or *tympanic membrane* into the middle ear, it is called *otitis media* for "middle," or *otitis interna* for "internal" if the disease is deep within the apparatus of the ear that controls balance.

Ear mites and bacterial and yeast infections are the most common causes of otitis externa. Ear mites are highly contagious insect parasites that are transmitted between dogs and cats. The bacterial and yeast infections begin when the ear is damaged by the self-trauma of scratching at the ear mites, or from bite wounds incurred during cat fights. Foxtails and other foreign bodies inside the canal irritate it, which irritates the cat, who shakes his head and scratches his face and ear to remove them.

Both malignant and benign tumors occur in the ears and associated structures. White cats are particularly prone to squamous cell carcinomas of the pinna from sun exposure. Although this cancer usually grows slowly and can be surgically removed, it tends to recur. Polyps grow up the eustachian tubes from the back of the throat and into the ear. Tumors obstruct the ear canal trapping moisture, and causing secondary infections with bacteria or yeast.

Bacterial infections and tumors that extend past the eardrum are responsible for otitis media and interna. These can progress into the brain. Some forms of otitis appear without any apparent cause. We say this otitis media and interna is *idiopathic.*

The clinical signs of otitis include headshaking, scratching, discharge from the canal, odor, a tilt of the head, unequal pupil size, unusual eye movement, and deafness. As the inflammation extends deeper and deeper toward the brain, the apparatus that controls balance can be damaged, and the cat may collapse or roll. A veterinarian uses an otoscope to examine the canal and tympanic membrane. If the cat is uncomfortable from pain, anesthesia is used. A bacterial culture or cytology smears are made to identify the infecting organism.

Paramount in the treatment of otitis is control of the underlying problem. If there are ear mites, they must be eliminated; polyps or other tumors must be resected, as they stand in the way of effective topical therapy. Oral and topical antibiotics and antifungals are used. The ear canal must be thoroughly flushed clean of pus and debris before beginning topicals. This may require anesthesia. See also page 74, Ear drops and ointments; page 85, Cleaning and flushing ears; page 120, Ear mites; and page 158, Vestibular disease.

P

Pneumothorax

The lungs and heart and all the blood vessels and lymph nodes necessary to support those vital organs are suspended inside the chest cavity or thorax. When a cat breathes in, the muscular diaphragm moves back and air passes through the airways all the way to the air sacs where oxygen is exchanged for carbon dioxide. This is made possible by the fact that there is a relative vacuum inside the thorax. No air leaks out of the lung tissue into the chest, otherwise the vacuum would be lost and the lungs could not expand as easily or fully. If the lung tissue ruptures, such as might happen in a fall, air immediately escapes into the chest cavity. With every inhalation, more air is pushed into the space around the lungs. This air cannot escape from the thorax.

The presence of free air in the chest cavity is called *pneumothorax.* This air takes up space and prevents the lungs from expanding. Portions of the lung or whole lobes can collapse. Pneumothorax can be detected on radiographs. These cats are in severe respiratory distress; the free air must be removed.

This is accomplished in a crisis by simply suctioning the air off with a large syringe and needle. The hole in the lung tissue usually closes over by itself. Depending upon the severity of the rent in the tissue, the chest may need to be tapped and the air removed several times before the hole seals. A device called a chest tube can be inserted between the ribs to allow for frequent suctioning if a lot of air is leaking. If the leak does not close on its own, it must be closed surgically or the damaged lobe removed.

Other causes of pneumothorax besides trauma include ruptured tumors, lung abscesses, or what we call *idiopathic causes*—that is, we can't identify the problem. Pneumothorax is very dangerous and these patients are very unstable. Pneumothorax due to trauma is usually not a problem once treated.

Pyometra

An infection of the uterus is called *pyometra.* Actually, this is a specific type of infection, one where there is a significant amount of pus that accumulates inside this organ. It is not very common in cats but is much more common in dogs. The uterus becomes infected by bacteria that arrive there either through the bloodstream from an infection somewhere else in the body, or by the movement of bacteria up the genital tract from the vagina and through the cervix. Once established, the bacteria infect the wall of the uterus. The body sends massive numbers of pus cells into the tissue to fight the infection. This causes an accumulation of pus similar to what happens when an abscess forms. The pus may drain from the uterus through the cervix. In this case, there is a foul odor and pus appears around the vulva. More often than that, the cervix remains closed and pus continues to accumulate and expand the uterus. Pyometra probably takes several weeks to develop to the point where the cat feels awful and loses her appetite, and becomes dehydrated, thin, and febrile. Unless the pus is draining out the vulva, there are no specific signs of pyometra.

Sometimes the enlarged uterus can be felt on physical examination or seen on radiographs. A complete blood count and chemistry panel are done to evaluate the patient to see if other organs have been affected by the infection.

The most realistic and humane treatment for pyometra in non-breeding cats is *ovariohysterectomy* or *spaying*. The infected, pus-filled uterus is removed, as are the ovaries. The cat is given antibiotics and fluids, usually intravenously. In cases where the infected uterus is draining out the vulva, a drug called a prostaglandin is sometimes given. This powerful drug causes the uterus to contract and empty. It can preserve the reproductive capabilities of a valuable breeding queen. Prostaglandins have considerable undesirable side effects. This therapeutic approach is not widely used in cats.

Pyometra is a serious illness with effects on many organ systems. The infection can spread to other tissues. The uterus can rupture, causing severe peritonitis or generalized infection throughout the abdominal cavity. Untreated, it is most likely to be fatal.

Pyothorax

An accumulation of pus inside the thorax or chest cavity is called pyothorax. *Pyo-* means pus. Most of the time, the cause of pyothorax is unknown. It is speculated that the bacteria that cause the infection that results in an outpouring of pus cells into the chest space come through the bloodstream from another source of infection in the body. Some examples would be a previous abscess or the gums, in cases of periodontal disease. Bacteria can be implanted by bullets from gunshot wounds. Fragments of bullets are often found incidentally on radiographs of animals and the owners are completely unaware that their pet has ever been shot. Penetrating and migrating foreign bodies like foxtail plant awns are notorious for causing these types of infection.

Cats with pyothorax can appear completely normal or may exhibit the types of signs one might expect with such a severe infection: fever, inappetence, dehydration, weakness, difficulty breathing, etc. The severity of the signs depends upon how slowly the infection progresses and how well the cat's immune system walls off the infection. Eventually the volume of pus becomes so great that the lungs can't expand very well and the cat breathes rapidly and with shallow breaths.

Pyothorax has a grave prognosis. Treatment is often unsuccessful. Remember that the hallmark treatment for abscesses—and that is essentially what this is—is drainage. It is very difficult to drain the chest cavity adequately. Sometimes the chest is irrigated or rinsed with a sterile antiseptic solution containing antibiotics. Antibiotics are also given orally and/or intravenously. A chest tube drain may be placed to allow continuous removal of the pus. Fluids are given intravenously. Treatment continues over several weeks. While I am not discouraging cat owners against treatment of pyothorax, I do believe that an owner should understand the risks, time, and expense involved in therapy.

R

Rabies

Rabies is an infectious disease of all warm-blooded animals, including humans. It is caused by several strains of virus that have a predilection for salivary glands and nerve tissue, especially the brain. Rabies is fatal in all animals except bats. Rabies can be transmitted to other animals through bat bites. Animals and people (spelunkers) who explore bat caves can become infected by breathing in air laden with virus contained in aerosolized bat urine.

Rabies in the wildlife population is called terrestrial rabies because the animals are on the ground. Epidemiologically speaking, terrestrial rabies is epidemic in raccoons, foxes, and skunks in large portions of the United States. Cats and other animals become exposed to rabies when bitten by these animals.

Because cats and other pets run free over the countryside, we don't know how often they actually come in contact with rabid animals. For the most part, people have much less of a chance of exposure to rabid wildlife. The whole point to mandatory rabies vaccination of dogs and cats is to create a protected barrier between us and the wildlife by vaccinating our pets who are at much greater risk.

Once rabies virus enters the body, it travels along nerves up towards the brain and salivary glands. In the brain, the virus causes seizures and dementia and eventually respiratory failure and death. It is always fatal in unvaccinated animals. The incubation period for rabies is usually about two weeks but can be up to six months; that is, it can take from two weeks to six months from the time it is bitten until an animal shows clinical signs of rabies. The animal can be perfectly normal until that time, but will, however, be able to transmit the virus to other animals. An unvaccinated, rabid cat who bites his owner can transmit the virus. That's why vaccinations are so important.

Rabies doesn't have to produce the furious dementia we witness in movies. Rabies has a "dumb" form where the animal becomes depressed, leading to coma. The dumb form of rabies is unlikely to be recognized as being rabies, making it much more dangerous. Unfortunately, cats have a tendency to exhibit the dumb form.

The clinical signs of rabies are viciousness, seizures, depression, paralysis, and other central nervous system abnormalities that can be seen with a lot of other diseases. The rabid animal usually dies within ten days of the onset of signs. Most veterinarians consider all cases of undiagnosed central nervous system disease as rabies until proven otherwise. If the owner, technician or doctor are bitten during an examination, or if

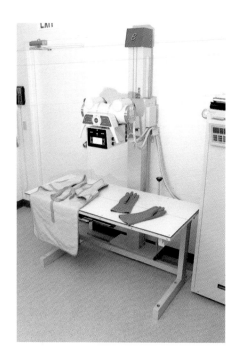

Modern x-ray machines produce high quality radiographs with minimal exposure times and little scatter radiation for the safety of the patient and the technicians. Personnel involved with x-rays wear lead aprons, gloves and thyroid shields, too.

saliva gets on cuts or injured skin, they can be infected.

The only way to confirm a case of rabies is by examination of the brain for the virus. This obviously requires euthanasia. There are state laws governing the handling of possible rabies cases. Depending upon the potential for animal exposure and the human risk, the law will range from quarantine to destroying the animal for examination of the brain. Your veterinarian and public health officials should be contacted for instructions.

Vaccinations are highly effective in preventing the disease even in the face of exposure. Without exception, cats should be vaccinated against rabies at 12 weeks of age and again one year later. If there are no state or town requirements for rabies vaccinations, at the very least cats should be given rabies boosters according to the manufacturer's recommendations.

Veterinarians will be familiar with the laws governing rabies vaccination in the face of potential exposure for your area. In recent years there have been more incidents of rabies in cats than in dogs in the United States.

Rodent Ulcer

See *Eosinophilic Granuloma Complex*

Ringworm

Contrary to what its name suggests, this is not a worm, but a fungal infection that occurs most often in kittens and occasionally in adult cats, especially Persian cats and related breeds. Many of these cats harbor the fungus in their hair follicles without a problem until they are stressed. At that time, the characteristic scaly patches of dry, hairless skin appear around the face and ears. Lesions develop on the paws because the cats wash their face and ears and spread the fungus to these locations. In some cases, the condition can involve the whole body and causes a patchy, moth-eaten appearance to the hair coat, or more rarely, scabs all over the back.

The diagnosis can either be made easily or require skin biopsies. The fungus infects the hair follicle. In about half the cases, ringworm fungus causes the hair to fluoresce apple green under an ultraviolet "black" light. It can also be identified on special preparations made from a few plucked hairs. Some uncharacteristic infections, i.e., the scabby kind, require biopsy to demonstrate the fungus. Cultures of the fungus can be helpful in determining what the species is and possibly where the cat picked it up. For instance, some ringworm fungus is found in the soil and is not that contagious.

There are a variety of treatments depending upon the number of lesions. Single hairless patches can be treated with topical antifungal creams. More extensive lesions require multiple baths with an antifungal shampoo and/or oral antifungal medications. Some of these medications cause abortion and birth defects in pregnant queens, so be sure to tell your veterinarian if your cat is pregnant. Treatment must continue for a number of weeks because most antifungals work by penetrating the hair shaft and interrupting the growth of the fungus, which is very slow.

Inadequate treatment and environmental contamination result in relapses. Some veterinarians recommend shaving a cat with severe ringworm to minimize the amount of fungus-containing fur that sheds into the environment. This fur must be removed from the environment as much as possible through vacuuming. A diluted bleach solution

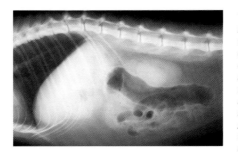

applied frequently to floors and other surfaces will kill the fungus.

This is a communicable disease. Children and immunosuppressed people have the greatest risk, but some healthy adults just get lucky. One unfortunate technician (and now veterinarian) friend of mine got ringworm three times and brought it home to all four of her cats, too.

The difference between the tissue density of bones, solid organs, fat and organs filled with air affect the passage of x-rays through the body and onto the x-ray film. These differences create an image such as this one. Visible on this radiograph are: some of the lung and heart, the liver, kidneys, portions of the intestinal tract, spine, ribs, and bladder.

S

Seizures (convulsions)

Seizures result when disorganized electrical activity in an area called a focus spreads to involve large portions of the brain that control consciousness, sensation, movement, and basic body functions. Borrowing the term from human medicine, most seizures in cats are described as the *grand mal* type. The cat loses consciousness and will not respond to the owner's voice or other stimuli. He collapses onto his side and alternately flexes and extends his limbs, or paddles them in the air as if to swim. Seizures cause the cat to defecate

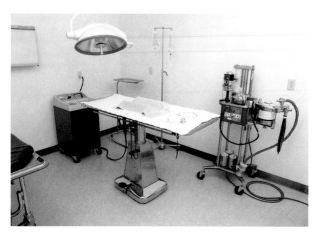

A surgical suite. From left to right: a gurney, light boxes for radiographs, pump for pediatric water-circulated heating pad on adjustable surgery table, overhead surgical light, instrument table, IV stand and gas anesthetic machine.

examination, laboratory and special tests can usually find those other diseases. Intracranial causes require involved and sometimes risky procedures such as electroencephalograms (EEGs), cerebrospinal fluid (CSF) taps, magnetic resonance imaging, and CAT scans.

Seizures resulting from extracranial causes can resolve if the primary disease is controlled. Seizures are also treatable with anticonvulsant medication. Intravenous diazepam (Valium) is used to stop the seizure. Phenobarbital is given once or twice a day to control recurrence of seizures caused by head trauma or epilepsy. Some seizures do not respond very well to anticonvulsant medications. Anticonvulsants do not completely eliminate epileptic seizures; most animals continue to have one or more now and again. Once anticonvulsant medications are started they should not be discontinued without veterinary supervision. Abruptly stopping these drugs can initiate status epilepticus.

A seizuring pet is very upsetting. My own dog Molly has an occasional seizure and even though I've seen hundreds of other animals' seizures, I was very alarmed when Molly had her first one. An owner whose cat is seizuring should not panic and stick something in the cat's mouth "to prevent him from swallowing his tongue." This isn't going to happen and the owner is likely to be bitten.

or urinate if the colon and bladder are full. He may tear, salivate, or vomit.

Most seizures last a few seconds or minutes. When a seizure lasts longer than five or so minutes and it appears that the cat isn't going to come out of it on his own, the seizure is called *status epilepticus*. Prolonged seizures cause damage to brain tissue. Status epilepticus is very harmful.

We divide the causes of seizures into two types: intracranial, or causes originating from inside the skull, and extracranial, or causes that originate outside the skull. Extracranial causes include poisons, organic diseases like kidney and liver failure, diabetes mellitus, and drug reactions. Intracranial causes would be things like head trauma, meningitis, brain tumors, epilepsy, and degenerative processes. It's much easier to rule out the extracranial causes of seizures than the intracranial ones. History, physical

The owner should call the veterinarian before rushing to the hospital. Drive carefully.

Sinusitis

Any upper respiratory disease is likely to involve the sinuses. Rhinotracheitis virus, Chlamydia, and calicivirus do the initial damage. Then bacteria that normally inhabit the nose and sinus passages begin to proliferate. The watery nasal discharge seen in the early stages of disease will change to a thick, cloudy mucus.

Sometimes sinusitis becomes chronic or recurrent. If there has been a lot of damage to the internal structures of the nose called *turbinates,* an important protective filtering mechanism has been lost. This is especially true in flat-faced breeds like Persians where the normal protective anatomy is less efficient. New bacterial or fungal invaders, especially the soil-borne fungus *Cryptococcoses*, can become established.

A deep-seated sinusitis is very difficult to treat. Long-term antibiotics and antifungals often fail to eliminate the infection. Surgical scraping and flushing of the sinuses has helped in some cases. Chronic nasal discharge suggests chronic sinusitis. Cancer of the nasal or sinus tissues appears identical to chronic sinusitis and must be considered in any refractory case.

T

Thromboembolism (Saddle thrombus, Systemic embolism)

Cats with heart disease are at risk for the spontaneous formation of blood clots, a condition called thromboembolism. When the clot or *thrombus* leaves the heart, it becomes lodged at some point along the circulation and cuts off the blood supply to the area nourished by that vessel.

The thromboembolism frequently recognized in cardiomyopathy occurs at the end of the aorta, the large artery that leaves the heart to supply blood to the whole body. It courses along the body wall just under the spine. Branches of the aorta exit along its path that ends as it forks into two branches called *iliac arteries*, one going to each hind limb.

It is here that thromboembolism most often occurs, at the iliac arteries. In the common vernacular, we call this a *saddle thrombus* because it conjures up an accurate visual image. The corollary event in human medicine might be a clot that lodges in the brain causing a stroke, or a clot lodging in a coronary artery of the heart causing a myocardial infarction (MI, heart attack).

As one might expect, the lack of blood supply to the hind limbs starves the tissues for oxygen and causes a build-up of waste products from tissues. These cats are in excruciating pain. They cannot use their legs to stand or walk. The legs are cold and there is no pulse in the vessel inside the legs. Toenails clipped very short don't bleed.

Thromboembolism treatment is divided into two parts: treatment for the acute or immediate condition, and long-term treatment. Acutely, these cats are given injections of heparin and low doses of aspirin orally to inhibit other clots from being formed. The heart disease must be stabilized. There have been several experimental programs evaluating the "clot buster" drugs used in humans with varying results.

In the long term, cats with thromboembolism are given aspirin and appropriate treatment for the heart disease. The prognosis is guarded. The iliac arteries can open up again or *recanalize* as the clot is removed. The cat will gradually recover sensation and use of the limbs. The clot may also get larger and extend for enough distance through the aorta to obstruct the renal arteries that supply the kidneys. This causes kidney failure and death. Despite aspirin and heparin therapy, more clots can form and obstruct other vital organs. Recurrence is highly likely. See also *Cardiomyopathy.*

U

Umbilical Hernia

The unborn kitten receives all of its nourishment from its mother through the umbilical blood vessels that connect the fetal circulation with the placenta. At the time of birth, the umbilical vessels constrict and retract as the kitten is freed from the placenta by the mother. The opening in the abdominal wall through which the fetal blood vessels pass closes at this time. Sometimes this opening doesn't close completely. A small amount of fat becomes trapped in the opening, creating a sac-like protrusion in the abdominal wall at the umbilicus or "belly button." This is called an umbilical hernia. If the opening in the abdominal wall is large, a piece of intestine can be trapped. Occasionally, the contents of this sac will fluctuate in and out as the contents shifts.

An umbilical hernia is usually of no consequence unless it is large or a piece of intestine does become incarcerated inside, in which case it is surgically repaired. Surgical repair is also done for cosmetic reasons at the time of ovariohysterectomy in female cats, or anytime in male cats.

V

Vestibular Disease

A neurologic disorder in cats, vestibular disease involves the nerves within the brain and middle ear that control balance. Many owners who witness their cats with this problem think the cat is having a stroke. In fact, when the brains of cats with vestibular disease are examined, no evidence of a blood clot (the cause of stroke) is found.

Vestibular disease comes on suddenly. In the mildest form there may only be a tilting of the head and abnormal eye movements. More likely the cat will fall to one side, roll, cry, and be unable to stand.

The diagnosis is made after ruling out infections and other problems with the middle ear or brain, or other organic diseases. A thorough examination of the ear canal and radiographs of the skull are done. With vestibular disease, the ear radiographs will look completely normal.

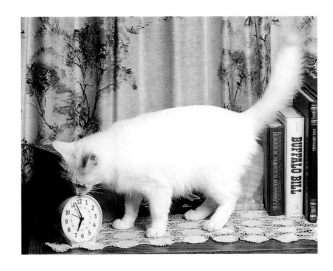

The cause for vestibular disease is not known and there is no treatment. Most cats recover on their own; however, there may be a permanent head tilt.

Appendix 1
Glossary of Medical Terms and Tests

This glossary contains selected tests with brief descriptions of why and how they're done and brief definitions of some anatomic terms. Like the rest of this book, it is not meant to be an all-inclusive discussion of feline diagnostic medicine, but rather a reference for you to turn to after your veterinarian has recommended a procedure. There are many laboratory tests that are not discussed because of space and complexity. These are the high points.

Acid-Base Balance A term that describes the body's ability to maintain the acidity or pH of the blood and tissue fluids close to normal. Mammals, as cats, dogs, and humans are, do this through complex buffering systems that involve the kidneys and lungs, salts like sodium bicarbonate, and proteins. Almost all diseases cause minor changes in the body pH that are rapidly corrected back to normal. This has little noticeable effect on the patient. However, during serious illnesses such as protracted vomiting and diarrhea, kidney dis-

ease, or traumatic injury, the buffering systems are severely taxed. Many of the salts and other buffering compounds may be lost from the body in the vomitus or diarrhea. The acid-base balance can be quite out of kilter for a long time. This becomes a complicating factor and can result in severe depression and even death. Fluid therapy is given to help restore the normal acid-base balance.

Allergy See *Hypersensitivity*.

Ascites An accumulation of fluid in the abdominal space. The fluid is produced during severe inflammation as in feline infectious peritonitis, or from heart disease, leakage of plasma from damaged blood vessels, or diseases that lower the amount of the protein called albumin in the blood. (Think of albumin as acting like a sponge holding plasma inside vessels.)

Azotemia A term that describes an excess of blood urea nitrogen.

Bacteriuria Bacteria present in the urine; this term is usually applied to patients who have an infection anywhere along the urinary tract from the kidneys to the bladder.

Baerman Fecal Test A method of analyzing feces for parasite larvae. Feces are mixed with water and put in a strainer that rests in a funnel fitted with a clamped piece of tubing to close off the bottom. A light is directed over the funnel. The warmth from the light stimulates the larvae to swim out of the fecal material and into the water in the funnel. After several hours of incubation, the larvae have sunk to the bottom. The clamp on the tubing is opened and a small amount of the solution is released from the funnel. Using a microscope, this solution is examined for larvae.

Barium Series (upper or lower G.I. series) A series of radiographs (x-rays) taken of the gastrointestinal tract using a material to provide contrast for comparison. For an upper G.I. series, barium or another similar contrast material is given by mouth, either alone or mixed with food. A series of radiographs are taken at different times so that the passage of contrast material can be followed as it moves through the system. The doctor evaluates the films for abnormal shapes, sizes, and thickness of the stomach and intestines; a change in the position of organs, movement, the time it takes for the material to move; and for foreign objects outlined by the barium. In a lower G.I. series, barium or other material is given by enema and several radiographs are taken to evaluate all of those parameters except for the elimination time. See also *Radiographs.*

Bilirubin A "waste" product produced from the breakdown of red blood cells. It is produced by the liver and excreted through the bile duct system into the intestines. Bilirubin is metabolized by the bacteria in the intestinal tract and then most of it is excreted with the feces. A small amount of bilirubin is normally found circulating in blood. Excessive levels often mean that there is some type of obstruction in the bile system associated with liver disease. When high levels of blood bilirubin "spill over" and are then detected in the urine, we say there is "bilirubinuria."

Biopsy A surgical procedure done to obtain tissue samples. There are many techniques and instruments available for collecting a biopsy, depending upon the tissue or organ that is being sampled. Once the tissue is collected, it is placed in a preservative such as formalin, alcohol, or liquid nitrogen for freezing. Formalin-fixed preservation is by far the most commonly used method. Once fixed, the tissues are embedded in paraffin wax and sliced into sections approximately 6 micrometers thick. The sections are adhered to glass slides and then stained with one of many diagnostic stains, depending upon what the doctor is looking for. Biopsies are obtained to detect cancer, infection, or any inflammatory process.

Bone Marrow Analysis A type of cytologic exam done to explain some abnormalities found in a complete blood count. The cells found in the bone marrow are responsible for producing red and white blood cells and platelets. A bone marrow analysis is performed when the patient has a profoundly low or very high red or white cell or platelet count. It is also done to see if the bone marrow is capable of producing new cells, or is producing too many cells of one particular type. Analysis also helps to determine if some forms of cancer have metastasized to the bone marrow. To do the analysis, a sample of marrow must be collected from one of several available sites: the hip, shoulder, or femur (long leg bone) are the usual places. The fur over the bone from which marrow is to be sampled is clipped, the skin antiseptically prepared as for surgery, and a local anesthetic is given. The doctor inserts a special needle through the overlying skin and muscle into the bone and then withdraws a few drops of marrow with a syringe. The samples are placed on glass slides, fixed, stained and evaluated along with a complete blood count. Most cats tolerate this procedure extremely well and do not require general anesthesia or an overnight hospitalization. See also *Cytologic examination*.

Bronchial Wash (transtracheal wash) A type of cytologic examination, this examines the secretions and cells within the air passages. There are two techniques; both require anesthesia in cats. A long, thin catheter is threaded into the trachea via a tube placed in the mouth. Alternatively, the catheter is passed between the tracheal rings. Either way, the catheter is threaded as far into the airways as possible, and a small amount of sterile saline (salt water) is instilled. The saline is immediately retrieved by aspirating with a syringe attached to the catheter. The material that is recovered is examined under a microscope. Sometimes it is cultured for bacteria or fungus. Bronchial washes are very useful in determining the cause of a cough and most respiratory diseases. See also *Cytology examination*.

BUN (Blood Urea Nitrogen, Serum Urea Nitrogen) A blood test that measures the waste product urea that comes from the metabolism of dietary protein. Urea is produced by the liver and then excreted by the kidneys. In normal cats, the amount of BUN is influenced to a limited degree by the amount of protein in food: The greater the amount of protein in the diet, the more nitrogen waste that the liver must change to urea for excretion by the kidneys. Normally functioning kidneys keep the amount of urea in the blood within a narrow low range, even with high-protein diets. When the amount of urea in the blood exceeds the capacity of the kidneys to excrete it, as in kidney disease or aging, the BUN value on a chemistry panel becomes elevated. More significantly, the patient does not feel well, acts depressed, may vomit, and frequently will not eat or drink. Other patients drink excessive amounts of water and as a result, void large volumes of urine.

Cataract A cloudy defect in the lens of the eye that prevents light from passing through to the retina.

Chemistry Panel A blood test, or more accurately, a group of tests done to evaluate organ function. A general chemistry panel can reveal information about the kidneys, liver, and endocrine systems, and how these organs affect the body's electrolytes (salt balance). A chemistry panel involves a series of chemical tests for substances in the blood that are normally present in small amounts, but either increase or decrease in amount when the above organs are diseased. Abnormal results are more significant than normal results: *A cat can have serious disease and have a perfectly normal chemistry panel due to the nature of the tests and the substances being analyzed.*

Coagulation Profiles A series of tests that evaluate the cat's blood-clotting ability. Several disorders will cause a decrease or increase in the tendency of blood to clot: some liver and gastrointestinal diseases, rodenticides like warfarin, and some blood disorders are examples.

Complete Blood Count (CBC) A blood test that determines several important characteristics of red and white blood cells by counting the numbers of each type of cell and by looking at their size, shape, appearance, and degree of staining. A CBC tells whether or not the cat is anemic, and if so, whether or not the bone marrow is responding to the anemia. A CBC measures the amount of protein and albumin in plasma, and looks to see if there are adequate numbers of platelets in the blood. In examining the color of the plasma, a CBC also identifies or confirms the condition of icterus or jaundice in a patient. A single CBC is like a snapshot; it reveals the status of the patient at one point in time. Several CBC's done over a period of days, weeks, or months to reveal trends are a much better evaluation of a patient.

Conjunctiva The delicate tissues that line the inside of the eyelids.

Cornea The clear front layer of the eye.

Cyanosis A bluish coloration of the gums, cyanosis tells us that there is an inadequate amount of oxygen in the blood. This could result from diseases in the lungs that prevent the exchange of carbon dioxide in the blood for oxygen. A defect in hemoglobin, the chemical in blood that carries oxygen, also causes cyanosis. Drugs like acetaminophen (Tylenol) cause defects in hemoglobin.

Cytologic Examination (cytology, exfoliative cytology) A study of the cells that make up a tissue or tumor using one of several collection techniques. Cells can be collected by aspiration (applying suction) with a fine gauge needle and syringe (fine-needle aspirate) or during a biopsy. After aspiration, the needle contents are expressed onto a clean glass slide. Biopsy specimens can be daubed or rolled on the slide before being dropped into formalin for histologic examination. Cells from the surface of the tissue biopsy adhere to the glass. After the slides air dry, they are fixed, stained, and examined with a microscope.

Fine-needle aspirates are nearly painless and can be done without anesthesia. Some cytology techniques require only light sedation. Because of this, cytologic examinations can yield a diagnosis with minimal investment of time and resources. They are not, however, always as accurate or informative as the histopathology performed on a biopsy specimen.

Dyspnea Difficult or labored breathing. Dyspnea will be apparent by an increase in the respiratory rate, an increase or decrease in the respiratory effort, and open-mouth breathing.

Electrocardiogram (ECG,EKG) A measurement of the electrical activity in the heart. An EKG measures the "strength" of the electrical current generated by specific *nodes* or pacemakers as it travels through the heart muscle, to cause that muscle to contract. The electrical impulse is measured by a machine that transforms it into a wave pattern on a screen or moving strip of paper. By examining the size and shape of the waves, the doctor can determine if the electrical impulses are moving properly through the heart. EKG's tell us how rapidly the node "fires" off an impulse and we compare that to the actual heartbeat. There should be one impulse per heartbeat. EKG's also tell us if the electrical impulse is being generated by the proper node or pacemaker. A cat can have very significant heart disease and have a perfectly normal EKG. EKG abnormalities can, however, be very helpful in determining the type of heart disease, but more importantly, the type of treatment that's needed.

Endemic A term used to describe when an infectious agent such as a virus or bacteria is present in a low percentage of a population of animals all the time. When the percentage increases well over what is normally present, the agent is said to be *epidemic*. For example, rabies virus is endemic in the wildlife population. Because the number of cases of rabies has increased dramatically in recent years, rabies is said to be epidemic in the eastern United States also.

Endoscopy Examination of a body cavity like the trachea and lower airways, or upper or lower gastrointestinal systems using a fiberoptic instrument called an endoscope. This is a long hoselike instrument with a flexible fiberoptic light source that can be snaked down the esophagus or similar structure. Endoscopes come in different diameters. The doctor looks through this instrument, like a flexible telescope, for close examination of structures and tissues. Endoscopes have a channel through which a tool can be fed to obtain biopsies. This procedure requires anesthesia.

Estrus The period of the reproductive cycle when a female cat is receptive to the tom and will mate and ovulate.

Exploratory A surgical procedure done when a doctor needs to examine internal organs and tissues visually in order to make a diagnosis or obtain a biopsy. When an exploratory surgery of the abdominal cavity is done, it is called a laparotomy. Exploratories can be done in any body cavity or on any diseased tissue. For example, draining wounds can be explored for thorns or other migrating foreign objects. Exploratories can confirm a diagnosis that is suggested but not quite confirmed by other laboratory tests. They are also important in the treatment of some conditions. An exploratory may by required to confirm that it is, in fact, a piece of rubber thong blocking your cat's intestinal tract that is causing unremitting vomiting and diarrhea. Once confirmed, the surgeon would, of course, take it out. (That is a true story!)

Febrile To have a fever.

Fecal Flotation The most common method for detecting intestinal parasites, a stool sample about the size of a nickel is put into a vial with a solution that causes the parasite eggs to float to the surface. A thin piece of glass called a coverslip is placed over the top of the vial. The vial is then left to sit for several minutes, or is spun in a centrifuge. The parasite eggs rise to the surface and adhere to the coverslip when it is lifted off the vial. The coverslip is then placed on a microscope slide and examined for parasite eggs.

FeLV Testing Screening tests to determine if a cat is infected with the feline leukemia virus. While the test results are reported as being either positive (infected) or negative (not infected), the results must be interpreted in light of how sensitive and how specific the test is that was used to detect the virus. You have to have a good understanding of the nature of feline leukemia virus as well.

Testing can be performed on either blood, tears, or saliva. Most testing is done right in the hospital using blood and one of several commercially available kits called an ELISA test. This test is very sensitive. It can pick up very early infections before the cat (or kitten) has even had a chance to mount an immune response to the virus. This cat will have a positive ELISA test because it is in an early stage of infection. If the cat's immune system responds effectively, the cat eliminates the virus from the body and the ELISA test will be negative eight weeks later. If the immune response is not effective in eliminating the virus, the results will almost always stay positive.

What happens if the cat's immune system doesn't eliminate the virus completely from the body, but only from the blood? Say the virus is hidden inside some cells in the bone marrow. Since the ELISA test is done on blood samples, the results of a second ELISA test could be negative on retesting. Perhaps these cats mounted an inadequate immune response to the virus, or it may just be the nature of the virus. Nonetheless, these cats are infected with the virus even though the test does not say so.

We call this a latent infection. Latency can explain why a cat with a negative FeLV test could revert to having a positive one later on, when the virus comes out of hiding and begins to circulate in the blood. Only then would it be detected on an ELISA test. Latency is only one example of why the doctor and the cat owner should not interpret FeLV test results as absolute.

Cats with two positive ELISA tests done eight weeks apart are likely to remain positive on subsequent tests. They should be considered to be infected with the virus and to be shedding that virus in blood, saliva, tears, and semen.

Once in a while, an ELISA test can be positive even if the cat isn't infected with feline leukemia virus. To eliminate the possibility of making a false positive diagnosis, a second type of FeLV test can be done called an IFA. This tests for the presence of the virus on the surface of white blood cells. It will only be positive if the virus has gone on to establish itself in the bone marrow of the cat. Cats with both a positive ELISA and IFA are unquestionably infected.

FIV Testing Screening tests to determine if a cat has been infected by the feline immunodeficiency virus and has mounted an immune response. Unlike the FeLV tests, FIV testing does not detect the virus itself, but rather the body's immune response to the virus by detecting the antibodies produced against it. Shortly after infection, the cat's immune system will respond to produce these antibodies. These cats will have a positive FIV test. The cat may go on to eliminate the virus from its body, or the virus may establish itself permanently. Typically, late in the infection when the cat's immune system is suppressed, those antibodies can no longer be produced. These cats will now have a negative FIV test, even though the cat is in fact infected. In a practical sense, if a cat is demonstrating the syndromes associated with FIV infection, one might be misled into thinking that this is *not* the root cause of the signs if one were to rely soley on the test results to make that judgment.

Foreign Body Any object, usually inanimate, that is found inside a body cavity or tissue. Common foreign bodies in small animals include small toys or socks inside the intestinal tract of puppies or strings in cats, or foxtail plant awns inside the ears and nose. Foreign bodies can be implanted in tissues, such as thorns lodged in the webs between the toes or BB pellets in muscle.

Fundus The innermost layer of the eye that includes the retina, the blood vessels that nourish it, the optic disc, and the tapetum. The fundus is examined using a handheld lens and a concentrated light source or an ophthalmoscope.

Glomerulus The portion of the kidney responsible for filtering blood of urea and other waste products.

Glucose Sugar, the primary fuel source for body tissues.

Glucosuria (glycosuria) Describes the presence of glucose in the urine. This can occur for short periods of time when a cat is under stress. Persistent glucosuria is a cardinal sign of diabetes mellitus in all domestic animals and humans.

Heinz Bodies Aggregates of abnormal (oxidized) hemoglobin found in red blood cells, they cause the red cells to be misshapen and fragile. They are easily identified on a CBC; the red blood cells with Heinz bodies have "noses"! Heinz bodies are normally found in small numbers in cats' blood and, for reasons not quite explained, sick cats tend to have a few more than normal. Large numbers of Heinz bodies can be caused by certain drugs and chemicals. Where cats are concerned, acetaminophen (Tylenol) ingestion is probably the most common cause. The chemical *propylene glycol* was a common additive to semimoist cat foods, giving them their characteristic texture. The FDA no longer allows this chemical to be used because it has been shown to cause the formation of Heinz bodies in red blood cells. In large numbers, Heinz bodies cause a severe anemia when these fragile red cells break down.

Hemoglobinuria Describes the presence of hemoglobin in urine. Hemoglobinuria almost always indicates that red blood cells have been destroyed or *lysed* in circulation and have released their hemoglobin. The hemoglobin is filtered by the kidneys and excreted in the urine. There can be many causes for red cell breakdown.

Hemolysis A breakdown of red blood cells, this occurs inside blood vessels or organs as a result of many diseases and some drugs. It can also occur naturally when blood is collected and stored prior to analysis, which can cause inaccuracies in some tests.

Hemothorax Blood within the chest cavity, hemothorax is usually a result of a ruptured blood vessel from trauma, such as might happen when a cat is hit by a car. Ruptured internal abscesses or tumors can also cause hemothorax. The rupture may seal on its own or require surgery to locate and ligate the vessel.

Hernia A prolapse or protrusion of an organ or tissue through an abnormal opening. Common hernias are diaphragmatic and umbilical.

History A chronological recount of the onset and progression of clinical signs associated with an illness. An example of a history might be: My cat began having diarrhea three weeks ago. In the beginning it only happened once a day and the stools were a little soft. Now he has diarrhea two or three times a day and it's like a cow pie and full of mucus. Yesterday he vomited.

Hypersensitivity (allergy) A pronounced and sometimes inappropriate response by the immune system. Hypersensitivity responses can occur during the natural course of a disease or with exposure to any chemical or drug. The reponse can also happen if the immune system begins to recognize a body's own tissues as being abnormal or even foreign to itself. There is technically more than one type of hypersensitivity response that the immune system can make and hypersensitivity and allergy are arguably not the same term to immunologists and medical doctors for all species. However, for the purposes of this book, I use the terms interchangeably.

Icterus Also termed jaundice, this describes the yellow discoloration to the skin and other tissues due to an accumulation of bile pigments. Cats with obstructive-type liver diseases frequently become icteric. The yellow coloration is easily seen in the white part of the eye (the sclera), along the gums, and in advanced cases, on the inside, hairless portion of the ears on light-skinned cats. The plasma and serum collected for blood analysis will also have an intensely yellow coloration.

Insulin One of the hormones responsible for regulating blood-sugar levels. Diabetes mellitus is a disease where cats or other animals do not produce enough insulin, or alternatively, cannot respond to the insulin they do produce. Without insulin, glucose or sugar cannot enter cells to be used for fuel. Insulin is produced by the pancreas.

Iris The colored portion of the eye that relaxes and contracts, changing the size of the pupil and thus the amount of light that passes to the retina.

Ketones An alternative fuel source for most tissues during periods of starvation. High levels of ketones in the blood also occur in diabetes mellitus. In both conditions, glucose or sugar is largely unavailable to tissues so the body turns to fat for energy. Ketones are a product of the metabolism of fat. High levels of ketones in the body is termed *ketosis.* One type of ketone is a substance called acetone. Animals with ketosis often have a characteristic odor of acetone (some nail polish removers are made of acetone) to their breath.

Ketonuria Refers to ketones being present in the urine. Ketones are not a normal component of urine and when detected, indicate that there are high levels in the blood and are now "spilling over."

Leukopenia A general term that describes a low number of white blood cells in circulation as determined by a CBC.

Lesion An abnormality in any structure. Skin lesions include crusts, pimples, bite wounds, etc. Eye lesions could include corneal ulcers, cataracts, or detached retinas. A heart lesion might be an enlarged chamber or an obstruction to the flow of blood, and so forth.

Lymphopenia A low number of lymphocytes in circulation. Lymphocytes are one type of white blood cell. They are derived from the bone marrow. They mature and are stored in several sites—bone marrow, lymph nodes, spleen, and thymus in young cats to name a few. Lymphopenia is commonly detected on a CBC and is due to stress, infection, inflammation, and some endocrine diseases.

Neurologic Examination An evaluation of the nervous system to determine whether a neurologic problem involves the brain, spinal cord, or the nerves that exit those organs. A neurologic exam tests the animal's ability to sense a stimulus like a pinch or prick, and to respond to the stimulus, as withdrawing a limb away from the prick. The previous example is a test of an animal's voluntary response. A neurologic exam also tests involuntary responses, such as like the change in size of the pupil to light and the knee-jerk reflex.

Neutropenia A low number of neutrophils in circulation. Neutrophils are another type of white blood cell that is produced in the bone marrow. They act as a first line of defense against infection and are an important player in the inflammatory response of the immune system. Neutropenia is detected on a CBC early in inflammation as the body's immune system calls them out of the bloodstream and into the site where they are needed. As the demand for neutrophils increases, the bone marrow responds by making more and the number of neutrophils in the blood will go back up. If the inflammation or infection is overwhelming, the bone marrow may not be able to keep up with the demand and the neutropenia will persist. This is a grave sign.

Neutrophilia The opposite of neutropenia, this term means there is a high number of neutrophils in circulation. When the demand for this white blood cell increases, the bone marrow is stimulated to produce more. This is reflected by an increase in the neutrophil count on a CBC. The magnitude of the increase over what would normally be circulating correlates roughly with the severity of the disease: Very high white-blood-cell counts usually mean that there is a severe inflammation somewhere in the body. For example, neutrophilia is common with pyometra.

Oliguria A term that describes scant urine production. This can occur for several reasons, including the acute kidney disease that occurs with antifreeze ingestion.

Optic Disc The site on the fundus where all the nerves from the retina come together to form the optic nerve. It appears as a whitish spot.

Perineum The area of the body under the tail and surrounding the anus and external genitalia.

Plasma The straw-colored fluid that suspends the cellular components of blood. It is rich in proteins, especially albumin and antibodies. Some transfusions are done using plasma rather than whole blood when the red blood cells are not necessary. It differs from serum, which is devoid of the clotting factors that are still present in plasma. Plasma is prepared by collecting blood into a collection vessel that contains an anticoagulant to prevent clotting. The blood is spun in a centrifuge. The cellular components like red and white cells will sink to the bottom and the plasma can be gently removed from the top.

Platelets A cell-like component of blood that is important in the formation of a clot. Platelets are produced by the bone marrow and occasionally by the spleen and liver.

Polydipsia Means excessive water consumption (drinking). Like polyuria, this is a sign of disease rather than a disease entity. Polydipsia is often difficult to document if a cat has more than one source of water. Gradual increases in water consumption are often missed by the owner, especially if the cat is reclusive. See page 180 for instructions on how to measure water consumption.

Polyuria Refers to excessive urine production. This is a sign of a disorder rather than a disease in itself. The list of possible causes is quite long, but in the cat the three main reasons for polyuria are kidney disease, hyperthyroidism, and diabetes mellitus. Other causes include excessive salt intake as with high salt diets, some drugs like corticosteroids, liver disease, and the polyuria seen after urinary obstruction in male cats. Polyuria will not be detected, of course, unless the cat uses a litterbox. Excessive urine production can lead to thirst and an increase in the amount of water a cat drinks. See *polydipsia*.

Proteinuria A term used to indicate that protein is present in urine in amounts greater than normal. Imagine the glomerulus as a kind of filter with small openings through which some substances like salts can pass. Most proteins are not normally allowed to pass through the glomerulus and into the urine because of their size. If the glomerulus becomes diseased, the filter openings can become larger and allow proteins to be lost in the urine. Protein loss in excess of the body's ability to replace it can result in severe wasting. Proteinuria can also occur with other diseases, notably a urinary tract infection.

Pruritic Itchy.

Pupil The elliptical opening in the iris that allows light to pass through to the retina.

Purulent Filled with or producing pus.

Radiographs (X-rays) Images created on film similar to a photograph, but made using x-ray energy instead of light. X-rays pass through tissues and create images on film on a scale from very black through gray to white, depending upon the tissue's density. Metal plates and pins, being very dense, do not allow x-rays to pass through. The x-rays do not react with the silver particles on the film and therefore the film looks white where the metal is. X-rays pass unimpeded through air, therefore x-rays that pass through the air next to the animal as it lies on the film plate react with the silver grains on the film. These areas will be black after developing. Lungs, muscle, fat, skin, hair, tendons, and organs will appear in gray scale depending upon the tissue density and thickness or whether there is air inside the organ. A radiologist evaluates films on the basis of the gray scale, size and position of organs, and presence or absence of structures or foreign objects. Special radiographic techniques can be used to outline organs. Air, barium, or other substances can be used for contrast in bladders and the gastrointestinal system. When motion-picture radiographs are taken it is called fluoroscopy. When radioactive isotopes are used instead of x-rays, it is called scintiradiography. This is sometimes done to identify tumors.

Retina The tissue lining the back of the eye that receives light and transmits it as a nerve impulse to the brain to create a visual image.

Serologic Testing A broad category of tests done on blood or the components of blood to determine whether an animal is infected or has been infected in the past with a particular disease-causing virus, bacteria, or fungi. Some examples of organisms for which serologic testing could be done include Feline Leukemia Virus (FeLV), Feline Infectious Peritonitis (FIP) Virus, Toxoplasma, *Cryptococcus;* in dogs, *Dirofilaria* (heartworm) and *Borrelia* (Lyme disease); and in people, the Human Immunodeficiency Virus (HIV). Some serologic tests look to see if the patient actually has the infection. Others look to see if the patient had it at one time and mounted an immune response (which may or may not have eliminated the infection, or the organism may still be lurking around the body somewhere). If that explanation sounds confusing, well, it can be. The results of many serologic tests require interpretation in light of the rest of what doctors like to call "the clinical picture." Only a few can definitively confirm that "he's got it." See also FeLV and FIV testing.

Skin Scrapings This is really a type of cytology exam, with a slightly different technique used to collect the sample. The surface of the skin, lesion, or sore is gently scraped with a scalpel blade or metal spatula. Some organisms like mange mites live deeply within the hair follicles, so the scraping must be deep enough to make the skin bleed. The material collected on the blade is gently smeared on a glass slide and is either covered with a drop of mineral oil or fixed and stained. The samples are examined under a microscope for potential causes of the lesions. Swabbing the ear canal and examining the debris for ear mites is another variation on this theme.

Steatorrhea Excessive fat in the stool, often associated with grayish diarrhea and a fouler-than-usual smell. Steatorrhea results from an inability to digest or absorb fats in the diet. This can be caused by diseases involving the liver, pancreas, or small intestine. Gastrointestinal infections with *Giardia* is an example.

Synovial Fluid Fluid located within joint spaces that is necessary for lubrication and nourishment of the joint surfaces and tissues.

Tapetum The shiny, reflective portion of the fundus that makes the cat's eye appear bright greenish yellow in the dark. Siamese cats and related breeds may not possess this structure. Their eyes will appear reddish under the same conditions.

T4 test A test that detects the amount of thyroid hormone circulating in the blood. High levels of T4 hormone are usually the result of a tumor in the thyroid gland or over-supplementation. Low levels of the hormone is associated with the condition of hypothyroidism which is uncommon in the cat.

Ultrasonography A diagnostic technique that uses sound waves to create images of organs and other structures on a screen. A transducer called a probe is placed on the skin. Some doctors will clip the fur and use a gel-like lubricant to insure good contact. High-frequency sound waves are emitted that are not audible to humans but can pass into tissues. The waves hit the tissues and bounce back to the probe. The information that is received is translated into a picture on a screen. Tissues will produce images that reflect the differences in densities between structures. The images are not the same as those created by x-rays. Ultrasonography shows the movement of organs and is especially useful in evaluating heart function and detecting pregnancies. Ultrasonography gives a three-dimensional assessment. It is noninvasive, unlike an exploratory. Some biopsies can be done guided by ultrasound. Ultrasound examinations do not require general anesthesia but may require light sedation in fractious patients.

Uremia See *Azotemia.*

Urinalysis (UA) Physical and chemical examination of a urine specimen. Urine is tested for the presence of several substances in abnormal amounts. The amount of salts in the urine is determined by measuring the specific gravity. The sample is concentrated using a centrifuge and the sediment is examined for red and white blood cells, crystals, and bacteria or other microorganisms that would suggest an infection anywhere along the urinary tract from the kidneys to the bladder, and possibly stones. The sediment is also examined for abnormal cells. A urinalysis gives information about several organ systems—liver, kidney, and endocrine.

Urine Casts Structures found in the urine sediment during a urinalysis that suggest damage to the tubules in the kidneys. Urine casts are largely made up of aggregates of sloughed cells and protein material. The number and type of casts can give an idea of the severity of the kidney damage and prognosis. Some drugs and poisons (antifreeze) cause casts to appear in urine.

Appendix 2
Useful Addresses and Literature

Veterinary Schools in the United States

Alabama
Auburn University
College of Veterinary Medicine
Auburn, AL 36849
(205) 844-4546

Tuskegee University
School of Veterinary Medicine
Tuskegee, AL 36088
(205) 727-8011

California
University of California
School of Veterinary Medicine
Davis, CA 95616
(916) 752-1360

Colorado
Colorado State University
College of Veterinary Medicine
and Biomedical Sciences
Ft. Collins, CO 80523
(303) 491-7051

Florida
University of Florida
College of Veterinary Medicine
Gainesville, FL 32610
(904) 392-4700

Georgia
University of Georgia
College of Veterinary Medicine
Athens, GA 30602
(706) 542-3461

Illinois
University of Illinois
College of Veterinary Medicine
2001 South Lincoln
Urbana, IL 61801
(217) 333-2760

Indiana
Purdue University
School of Veterinary Medicine
1240 Lynn Hall
West Lafayette, IN 47907
(317) 494-7607

Iowa
Iowa State University
College of Veterinary Medicine
Ames, IA 50011
(515) 294-1242

Kansas

Kansas State University
College of Veterinary Medicine
Manhattan, KS 66506
(913) 532-6011

Louisiana

Louisiana State University
School of Veterinary Medicine
Baton Rouge, LA 70803
(504) 346-3200

Massachusetts

Tufts University
School of Veterinary Medicine
200 Westboro Road
North Grafton, MA 01536
(508) 839-5302

Michigan

Michigan State University
College of Veterinary Medicine
East Lansing, MI 48824
(517) 355-6509

Minnesota

The University of Minnesota
College of Veterinary Medicine
St. Paul, MN 55108
(612) 624-9227

Mississippi

Mississippi State University
College of Veterinary Medicine
Mississippi State, MS 39762
(601) 325-3432

Missouri

University of Missouri
College of Veterinary Medicine
Columbia, MO 65211
(314) 882-3877

New York

Cornell University
College of Veterinary Medicine
Ithaca, NY 14853
(607) 253-3000

North Carolina

North Carolina State University
College of Veterinary Medicine
4700 Hillsborough Street
Raleigh, NC 27606
(919) 829-4200

Ohio

The Ohio State University
College of Veterinary Medicine
Columbus, OH 43210
(614) 292-1171

Oklahoma

Oklahoma State University
College of Veterinary Medicine
Stillwater, OK 74078
(405) 744-6648

Oregon

College of Veterinary Medicine
at Oregon State University
Corvallis, OR 97331
(503) 737-2141

Pennsylvania

University of Pennsylvania
School of Veterinary Medicine
3800 Spruce Street
Philadelphia, PA 19104
(215) 898-5438

Tennessee

University of Tennessee
College of Veterinary Medicine
Knoxville, TN 37901
(615) 974-7262

Texas
Texas A&M University
College of Veterinary Medicine
College Station, TX 77843
(409) 845-5051

Virginia
Virginia Tech and
University of Maryland
Virginia-Maryland Regional College
of Veterinary Medicine
Blacksburg, VA 24061
(703) 231-7666

Washington
Washington State University
College of Veterinary Medicine
Pullman, WA 99164
(509) 335-9515

West Virginia
Board of Veterinary Medicine
1900 Kanawha Blvd East
Charleston, WV 25303

Wisconsin
The University of
Wisconsin-Madison
School of Veterinary Medicine
Madison, WI 53706
(608) 263-6716

Wyoming
Board of Veterinary Medicine
Herschler Building
Cheyenne, WY 82002

For schools and teaching hospitals outside of the United States contact the AVMA at:

American Veterinary
Medical Association
1931 North Meacham Road
Suite 100
Schaumburg, IL 60173
(800) 248-2862

Two Large Private Hospitals:
Angell Memorial Animal Hospital
350 South Huntington Avenue
Boston, MA 02130
(617) 522-7400

Animal Medical Center
510 East 62nd Street
New York, NY 10021
(212) 838-8100

Some Specialty Boards in Veterinary Medicine
Anesthesiology
Cardiology
Dentistry
Dermatology
Emergency and Critical Care
Internal Medicine
Neurology
Nutrition
Oncology
Ophthalmology
Pathology
Surgery
Radiology
Reproduction

Veterinary Schools in Canada

University of Montreal
Faculty of Veterinary Medicine
Saint Hyacinthe
Quebec, Canada J2S 7C6

Ontario Veterinary Collete
University of Guelph
Guelph, Ontario,
Canada N1G 2W1

University of Prince Edward Island
Atlantic Veterinary College
Charlottetown, Prince
Edward Island,
Canada C1A 4P3

University of Saskatchewan
Western College of Veterinary
Medicine
Saskatoon, Saskatchewan,
Canda S7N 0W0
(306) 966-7103

Cat Clubs

The American Cat Association
8101 Katherine Avenue
Panorama City, CA 91402
(818) 782-6080

American Cat Fancier's Association
P.O. Box 203
Point Lookout, MO 65726
(417) 334-5430

Canadian Cat Association
52 Dean Street
Brampton, ON L6W 1M6

The Cat Fancier's
Association, Inc.
1805 Atlantic Avenue
P.O. Box 1005
Manasquan, NJ 08736
(908) 528-9797

The International Cat
Association
P.O. Box 2684
Harlingen, TX 78551
(210) 428-8046

Associations Devoted to Animal Welfare and/or Disease Research

American Animal Hospital
Association
12575 West Bayaud Avenue
P.O. Box 150899
Denver, CO 80215
(303) 986-2800

American Association of
Feline Practitioners
7007 Wyoming NE, Suite E-1
Albuquerque, NM 87109

The American Society for the
Prevention of Cruelty to Animals
424 East 92nd Street
New York, NY 10128
(212) 876-7700

American Veterinary Medical
Association
1931 N. Meacham Rd., Ste. 100
Schaumburg, IL 60173
(800) 248-2862

Canadian Veterinary Medical
Association
339 Booth Street
Ottawa, Ontario, Canada, K1R 7K1
(613) 236-1162

Cornell Feline Health Center,
Cornell University, College of
Veterinary Medicine
Ithaca, NY 14853
(607) 253-3414

Delta Society
Century Building, Third Floor
321 Burnett Avenue South
Renton, WA 98055
(206) 226-7357

The Humane Society of
the United States
2100 L Street NW
Washington, DC 20037
(202) 452-1100

Massachusetts Society
for the Prevention of Cruelty
to Animals
350 South Huntington Avenue
Boston, MA 02130
(617) 522-7400

Morris Animal Foundation
45 Inverness Drive East
Englewood, CO 80112
(303) 790-2345

Publications Related to Feline Health Topics

Catnip A newsletter for caring cat owners, published monthly by Tufts University School of Veterinary Medicine. Subscriptions cost $24 per year. For information write or call: Catnip, P.O. Box 420014, Palm Coast, FL 32142, 1-800-829-0926

Perspective on Cats A newsletter for cat fanciers from Cornell University and the Cornell Feline Health Center. Contact the Cornell Feline Health Center, 618 VRT, Ithaca, NY 14853 for information.

Other publications:

Animals Magazine is published bimonthly by the Massachusetts Society for the Prevention of Cruelty to Animals, 350 South Huntington Ave, Boston, MA 02130. Subscriptions cost $19.94 per year. Call 1-800-998-0797.

CATS Magazine is published monthly by CATS Magazine, Inc. 2750-A South Ridgewood Ave., South Daytona, FL 32119. Subscriptions cost $18.97 ($24.97 for Exhibitors Edition) for one year.

Popular Cats is published bimonthly by Harris Publications, 1115 Broadway, New York, NY 10010. Subscriptions cost $9.97 per year for six issues.

Useful Books

Behrend, K., and Wegler, M. *The Complete Book of Cat Care: How to Raise a Happy and Healthy Cat.* Barron's Educational Series, Inc., Hauppauge, 1991.

Caras, Roger. *A Cat Is Watching: A Look At the Way Cats See Us.* Simon and Schuster, New York, 1989.

Frye, Fredric, L. *First Aid for Your Cat.* Barron's Educational Series, Inc., Hauppauge, 1987.

Maggitti, Phil. *Guide to a Well-Behaved Cat.* Barron's Educational Series, Inc., Hauppauge, 1993.

McDonough, Dr. Susan. *The Complete Book of Questions and Answers Cat Owners Ask Their Vet.* Running Press, Philadelphia, 1980.

Morris, Desmond. *Catwatching.* Crown Publishers, Inc., New York, 1986.

Siegal, Mordecai (ed). *Cornell Book of Cats: A Comprehensive Medical Reference for Every Cat and Kitten* by the Faculty and Staff of the Cornell Feline Health Center, Cornell University. Villard Books, New York, 1992.

Fiction:

Amory, Cleveland. *The Cat Who Came for Christmas.* Little, Brown and Company, Boston. 1987.

Camuti, Dr. Louis. *All My Patients Are Under the Bed.* Simon and Schuster, New York, 1980.

Mooney, Samantha. *Snowflake in My Hand.* Delacorte Press, New York, 1989.

Appendix 3
How to Measure Water Consumption

To measure the amount of water that your cat drinks in a 24-hour time period, start by filling the bowl with a known quantity of water:

Day 1: 8 AM

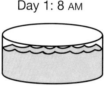

16 oz. (480 ml)

At about the same time the next day, measure the amount of water that is left in the bowl:

Day 2: 8 AM

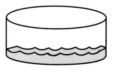

2 oz. (60 ml)

The difference between what you started with and what was left is the amount of water your cat drank. 16 oz. – 2 oz. = 14 oz. (480 ml – 60 ml = 420 ml).

If you have to refill the bowl during the day, be sure to measure and add together all the amounts that you added.

Day 1: 8 AM

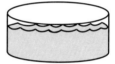

Day 1: 6 PM

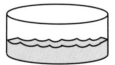

Day 2: 8 AM

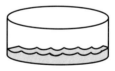

16 oz. (480 ml) + 8 oz. (240 ml) – 2 oz. (60 ml) = 22 oz. (660 ml)

Write down the amount of water that your cat drinks each day on your calendar.

Index